CONTENTS

Introduction	1
Preparing for PA school	2
What to expect	7
Didactic year	14
Clinical Year	51
Earning your master's	76
I've graduated. Now what?	78
Conclusion	83

INTRODUCTION

You got into PA school!! Woo-Hoo!! Congrats to you!! Getting into PA school is no easy feat and I know that you worked really, really hard to get to this point. Clearly, you are a smart, capable individual who is not afraid to roll up those sleeves and get down to business. And that's a good thing because … this is just the beginning. You are about to experience an experience like no other: a two(ish) year whirlwind of learning and training that will knock you down, pick you back up and send you on your way to your dream career. But before that, there are some things you should know and some things you should do that will make this transition period a bit smoother.

PREPARING FOR PA SCHOOL

Now that the excitement of getting into PA school has begun to fade and give way to anticipation, nervousness, questions and doubt, there are some things that you should do before school starts. First, take some time off. That's right. Don't try to get ahead by taking an online Intro to Pathophysiology course or by going over your undergrad anatomy notes. Instead, do something that relaxes you and puts you in a good headspace. There is plenty of time for learning and guess what? You will spend the majority of your time doing just that soon enough. For now, read a great book series, have a movie marathon, paint a masterpiece, hike a couple of mountains, yarn bomb your neighborhood park (with permission, of course!), go on a dessert tour, sneak away for a weekend of golf - whatever it is that brings you joy, do that. Make time to do some stuff that you really love to do with the people who you really love being with and make great memories with them. Believe me, being able to think back on those good times will get you through the tough times ahead.

Let your family know that you will pretty much be unavailable for the next two or so years. Really. And prepare yourself for that, as well; this is nothing like undergrad. Tell all of your loved ones how much you love and appreciate them and explain to them that you really need their support and understanding as you head off to school. Because once you are in school, school is pretty much all you will do. Free time is minimal as you navigate the rigorous schedule and academic demands of graduate study. This is especially true in the beginning as you acclimate and find your footing. Knowing that all is well on the home front and that your loved ones will be there, waiting for you on the other side, is a nice feeling.

Tie up any loose ends

Do your best to settle any issues outside of PA school before you begin PA school. Try really hard to not bring any extra baggage. Take care of any outstanding debts or responsibilities, get a clean bill of health from your doctor, let your dentist polish your pearly whites, make sure you have your prescriptions and figure out how you will get from here to there. Give your notice at your job and let your landlord know when you'll be moving out. If you are staying at home, make sure you have a quiet space all to yourself where you can do what you need to do without being interrupted. And finally, let go of what needs letting go of, whether it is a toxic relationship, negative thoughts, time-wasting habits, or anything else that will distract you from your goal.

Take care of any pre-program requirements

Check with your program to see what you need to do before the first day of school. Read and re-read your welcome packet. Make a list of all the things you need to do before you step foot onto campus. If you need a laptop, make sure that you have one that meets the requirements set forth by the school. Don't bring the rickety old hand-me-down you got from your sister. If you need to download software, do that. And if you have trouble with it, get in touch with someone from IT to help you. Make sure that you have all of the necessary medical documentation, including proof of vaccinations. Some programs require completion of a medical terminology or anatomy survey prior to the start of school. Make sure that these things are done well before their due dates. Most students require some sort of financial aid to pay for school. Check in with the financial aid office to make sure that everything is in order.

Attendance policy

Familiarize yourself with the attendance policy. Each school has different policies. One program may allow an excused absence so that you can be the best man at your brother's wedding, but only if they are aware of the event up front, while other programs may not allow for it at all. Also, more than likely you will not be excused from class so that you can go to Aunt Gertrude's retirement party or Cousin Becky's baby shower. Getting permission to leave school Thursday and Friday to go to a bachelorette in St. Lucia is highly unlikely. You have been accepted into PA school and you are expected to go to PA school – all of it. This is your life for the next two years or so. Prepare for that mentally. Be ready to say no to a lot of stuff that you really want to say yes to. And yes, this really stinks. But, in the grand scheme of things, this is only two years of your life. And you have made a commitment.

Figure out your living situation

Many of you will be moving away to go to PA school. Most campuses do not offer graduate housing, so finding a place to live is very important. Get your living situation in order well before PA school starts. You will be stressed enough with the idea of PA school and hanging out with new people, not to mention good ole performance anxiety, imposter syndrome, etc., etc. Don't pile rushing around to make living arrangements onto that ever-growing huge heap of stress. Do your research and become familiar with the neighborhoods near the school. Pay attention to details like safety, crime rates, walkability, public transportation, and proximity to the school. PA school typically starts early in the morning and can go late into the evening. The shorter the commute, the better, in most cases. Speaking of commute, will you have a car? What is the parking situation on campus? If you don't have a car, how will you get to school? Is your apartment within walking distance? Is it a safe neighborhood to walk in? How will you carry your laptop, books, equipment, lunch, etc.? Is there public transportation and does it run the times that you need to be publicly transported? What is the closest, safest neighborhood that you can afford? Are you willing to share with a roommate? These are all questions that, if answered before you arrive, will make things much easier for you.

As you probably know, there are many pre-PA forums out there that make it easy to connect with other first year PA students in your program. This is a great place to ask questions, compare notes, commiserate, celebrate, and possibly find a roommate. More often than not, one of those classmates will be from the area and will be a good resource for all things local. Additionally, most programs set up social media accounts for the new students so that they can get to know each other. Participate!

If you can, arrive at least a week or two before school starts to get your living arrangements in order. Get settled in and start looking around. Meet up with classmates. Check out the area. Most programs sponsor meet and greets and mentoring programs with the second-year students, who organize all sorts of fun get-to-know-each other activities. At our program, for example, we have a citywide scavenger hunt that hits all the highlights of where to eat, where to shop, where to relax, where to work out and other points of interest. Take advantage of these activities! Find yourself a cute little coffee shop where you can go to study. Discover the safest running trails. Find that great vegan restaurant that delivers. Find your footing. The more familiar and comfortable you are with your new surroundings, the easier the transition will be.

Make your space homey and comfortable and, if you are living with someone else, negotiate the ground rules early on so that you and your roommate have clear expectations of one another. Most importantly, though, pause for a minute to just take it all in: You are about to start PA school. Huge accomplishment!!

WHAT TO EXPECT

Now, if you are like most of the students who are accepted into PA school, undergrad was a breeze. Well, maybe not a breeze, but I bet it's safe to say that you did pretty well. You probably worked really hard to earn all of those A's and you're probably used to doing well - maybe even being at the top of your class. And that's great. You should be proud of that. But be warned, PA school is nothing like undergrad. Nothing. You will struggle. Yes, you. You will struggle. You will be overwhelmed. You will doubt yourself and wonder if you've got what it takes. You may even fail something for the first time. And that's ok. That's all normal. PA school is nothing like anything you have experienced. It has been compared to drinking water from a fire hose. The huge volume of material that you are expected to master and the pace with which that mastery is expected is a shock to the system. The good news, though, is that everyone else is in the same boat. Your classmates have had similar successes and they are going to have the same doubts, fears, and perceived failures as you. You are in this together. Which leads me to ….

Classmates

Do Not Compare Yourself To Your Classmates.

You all have different strengths, weaknesses, talents, and abilities. My mom used to tell me that there will always be someone smarter, funnier, prettier, and taller than me. That is true for you, too. While you may shine in one area, someone else is the star somewhere else. Do not turn your classmates into your competition. Celebrate their victories, help them with their struggles and, above all else, lean into your unique experience because, believe it or not, you all have different things to learn. I am not talking about curriculum here. I am talking about life lessons and skills that *you* need to make *you* the best PA *you* can be. You have your own path to PA-C that is ripe with *your own lessons*. Lessons that, for whatever reason, you need to learn. That's why you are experiencing what you are experiencing. Every struggle is an opportunity for growth if you are open to the process. Perhaps you need to learn humility or the importance of collaboration. Maybe you need to learn how to laugh at yourself or loosen up. Or maybe you needed to really master that neuro exam because 5 years from now there will be a patient with an undiagnosed brain tumor who has signs and symptoms that are so subtle that only a practitioner who has practiced the neuro exam over and over and over again, as you had to do, can pick up on them and guess what? She's the next patient on your schedule. I don't know what the lesson is for you and you might not know right away, either, but there is a lesson. Specifically put there for you. Be open to learning from your mistakes, shortcomings, and failures. This is the safe time to do that. And don't worry about who is at the top of the class (or the bottom for that matter – unless you are in a position to help in any way). You do you. Do the best you can and help out when able, but don't compare.

Remember how I was saying that you probably excelled in undergrad? Well, if you happen to be a student who had, shall we say, some hiccups along the way in your undergrad career and just barely met the GPA requirements to be considered for PA school, don't doubt yourself now. You got in, just the same as the kid sitting next to you with the perfect GPA, shining recommendations and exceptional volunteer experiences got in. You earned your spot fair and square. Lean into that and believe in yourself.

Find Your Tribe

Find the people who will be there for you and with you throughout this crazy whirlwind of an experience. Having someone in your corner who you can laugh and cry with, who you can turn to for help and who you can depend on for letting off steam is crucial. Your circle can be wide or it can be small. It doesn't matter, as long as they are *your* people. And don't worry you will find your people. Having someone to look forward to seeing every day – yes, every day – just makes the whole process that much easier. I was lucky. I found my people early on and am so incredibly grateful for them. I look back on my time in PA school with such fondness. Sure, it was super hard and overwhelming at times. Yeah, I spent the majority of my time studying and prepping and sitting in class, but when I look back on it, I don't so much remember the work itself. What I remember is the time spent with my friends; those people who understood and knew exactly what I was going through like no one else. As supportive as my family was, nothing came close to the support from my people. Suppressing deliriously silly giggles during excruciatingly long lectures, settling into long comfortable silences during study sessions, having deep meaningful conversations over the rare beer and knowing what is needed from each other without needing to say a word; that is stuff like that that gets you through. It is stuff like that that you remember. Take a moment to cherish your tribe.

Find Your Soulmate?

Most people advise against dating a classmate, mostly because dating is a distraction and PA school is hard enough even without extra distractions. Think about new love – it's all giddy happiness filled with hearts and rainbows. Essentially, your head is in the clouds when it should be in the books. This in and of itself is distracting, but if things go bad, it can go really bad. I'd say just avoid the drama and distraction and stick to the task at hand. As a student, your focus should be on your studies, not on how cute her butt looks in those yoga pants or how dreamy his eyes are. That being said, you are an adult who is capable of making adult decisions. Just make sure that the decisions that you make are in your best interest and know that true love will still be true love after you walk across that graduation stage.

Be prepared for the possibility of failure

At some point in your PA school career, you will do poorly on a test or an assessment or a project. Trust me, you will. We all do and we all have. Learn what you can from the experience and move on. Don't doubt whether or not you belong there. Don't let it shake your confidence. Give yourself 5 minutes to wallow in all of those ugly feelings of doubt, self-pity, blame, anger, sadness, embarrassment and whatever else you may be feeling and then let it go. Let it go so that you can reflect on what happened and figure out where you went wrong. Maybe you were trying out a new study technique that didn't work for you or maybe you didn't take very good care of yourself for the couple of days leading up to the exam. Maybe you had some personal stuff going on or maybe you did so well on the last exam that you thought you could breeze through this one without working quite as hard. Or, perhaps you simply had difficulty grasping the big concepts. Whatever the situation, there is a reason that you did poorly (hint: the reason is not that your professor sucks). It is your job to figure out what happened so that you can make the necessary changes and adjustments that will ensure your success the next time around.

If it is a matter of understanding concepts, try to pinpoint what is giving you difficulty, see if you can figure it out and then go see your professors for help. That is why they are there. They want you to succeed and they are happy to do their part in helping you in your success.

Thankfully, repetition is built into the curriculum. For example, if you didn't quite understand in Pharmacology why you use Cefazolin for cellulitis, you get the chance to revisit the subject in the dermatology and infectious disease portions of your clinical medicine courses. Oh yeah, and you should see it at least a couple of times in clinical year.

Take care of yourself

Hard work, dedication and time management are all very important ingredients in the recipe for success and we will touch on them, but not just yet. What I want to focus on at this point is self-care. I cannot overemphasize just how important it is to take care of yourself, both mentally and physically. Nourish your body and mind with a healthy diet filled with fruits, vegetables, and whole grains. Although processed foods are quick and easy and sugary foods give a quick boost of energy, in the long run, they sap your energy, kill your motivation, and bring down your mood. You've heard that exercise is nature's anti-depressant? Who wouldn't want to get in on some of that? Seriously, though, daily exercise boosts your energy and stamina and helps you sleep better at night. If you have trouble sleeping, there are some changes that you can make to your environment that can help. Make sure that your room is nice and dark and a little on the cool side. If you have a herd of elephants living above you, get yourself some noise-cancelling headphones. Reserve your bed for sleeping only – that means no studying or web surfing. In fact, you should put down all blue-light emitting gadgets about an hour before bedtime and you should go to bed at roughly the same time each night. Unless you are one of those rare people who can get by on little sleep, you should aim for at least seven hours nightly.

Self-care

PA school can be super stressful. In addition to eating well, exercising regularly and prioritizing sleep, it is important to take time for self-care activities. I know that the idea of taking time to indulge in a stroll through the woods or sitting down to watch your favorite TV show seems counterintuitive, especially after I prattled on and on about how hard PA school is, but it is not. It is necessary for your well-being. We all need time to take a step back and reset. You will need to stay in touch with who you are outside of school in order to perform at your best. As an example, I had a very bright, capable student who was struggling academically. After some reflection, she realized that she was spending every waking minute studying or thinking about studying or worrying about studying or trying not to worry about studying. Her entire life had been shrunken down around school and she shut out something that had always brought her joy: dancing. Ballet had been a huge part of her life until she started PA school because she stopped dancing so that she could focus all of her attention on studying. Sounds logical, right? On the surface, sure. But looking at it a little more closely, she realized that eliminating something that had been such a big part of her life and, in fact, her identity, was a mistake. When she looked at it that way, she knew that denying herself the joy of dance was hurting her – and her grades. Once she reincorporated dance into her life, her grades improved. She wasn't dancing nearly as much as she used to, but it was just enough to bring a sense of balance. With that, she relaxed into her studies and saw improvement in her grades. From there, she flourished. The point is, continue to do what you love. If there is something in your life that lifts your spirits, replenishes your soul, and makes you feel good about yourself, make sure that you make space for it in your life as a PA student. You probably cannot dedicate as much time to it, but you can dedicate some amount of time to it and sometimes doing that makes all the difference.

Helpful hint: seek out professional help if you feel that your mental health is at risk. If you have a known mental health issue, make sure that you continue whatever therapeutic interventions you have in place or make sure that you establish care at the school. There is no shame in asking for help. In fact, it is encouraged. Doing so shows maturity, self-awareness, and bravery. Talk with your advisor or other trusted faculty member and use the resources that are available to you so that you can be the best you that you can be during this time.

DIDACTIC YEAR

The goal of didactic year is also its biggest challenge: prepare you for clinical rotations, all in twelve short months. Wait, twelve months is short? Yup. You'll know soon enough. Medicine is a huge subject and there is sooo much for you to learn before you step foot on a clinical site. Take a moment. Take a breath. You've got this.

Time management

PA school has a lot of moving parts. It is not unusual to find yourself studying for a lab practical, prepping for an exam, reading for journal club, finishing up a paper and working on a group project all in one week. A little planning is the key to successful time management. To-do lists, a master calendar and detailed weekly schedules help you keep track of all of those moving parts and help you figure out how to best use your time. I would highly recommend getting a monthly calendar, electronic or paper, and something separate that you can use to keep track of your daily, weekly, and monthly goals and responsibilities. Schedule everything from your to-do lists and all of your due dates onto your calendar and cross them off as they are completed. Take a peek at your calendar and schedule every day and add any new items that pop up on your to-do lists. The more well-organized your approach, the less stress you will have around your day-to-day activities. And guess what? The less stress you have, the better you do.

Make A Schedule

Take the time to sit down and plan out your week. Make that task part of your weekly schedule. Use the class schedule provided by your program to block off the times that you will be in class. You can probably print out the schedule and build the rest of your week around that. Don't forget to incorporate travel time, to and from school, especially if your commute is on the longer side. Next, schedule some down time every day. Even if it is just 10 minutes, put it on the schedule. Make time, as well, for tasky things that you have to get done in order to function, such as meal prepping, apartment cleaning, laundry washing and whatever else you need to do to keep things smoothly running. Now, grab your syllabus and figure out how much studying you need to do and where you can fit it into the schedule. I would suggest that you write a list of all of your responsibilities for that week, estimate how long it will take you to accomplish them and them start plugging them into the empty spaces on your schedule. Whatever you write on that schedule, you do. Commit to that now because without action and follow through, all of this is a meaningless waste of time.

As you create your weekly schedule, keep in mind any short- or long-term projects that are on the horizon. I would figure out all of the steps that you need to complete those tasks, estimate how long it will take you to accomplish each step and, working backward from the due date, determine when you need to start working on them. Why all the fuss about this? What's the big idea? Well, we have tendency to wait until the last minute to finish a task. This fact illustrates Parkinson's law, which states that work expands to fill the time allowed for completion of a task. Meaning, if your paper on the History of the PA Profession, for example, is due in a month, you just might languish for three and a half weeks, thinking that you have plenty of time left, only to find yourselves scrambling and hustling at the end, trying to get your finished paper handed in on time. A good strategy to avoid this is to create mini-deadlines for each step and stick to that schedule instead of focusing on the oh-so-far-away due-in-one-month deadline. When writing that history of the PA profession, for example, schedule an outline deadline, a research deadline, a first draft deadline, etc. This approach is especially helpful in your second year when you will be expected to write your Capstone or thesis paper.

Helpful hint: outlining different responsibilities in different colored highlighter – red for class time, blue for downtime, green for getting other stuff done, orange for study time – gives a nice visual of how you will spend your time.

Establish A Routine

We are creatures of habit. Our brains make habits out of repeated activities so that we can easily do them again and again without much thought; things like riding a bike, driving a car, turning the light switch on when we walk into a dark room, etc., are all habits formed through repetition. That is the brain's way of maximizing its power. We can take advantage of that.

Think of habit formation like organizing your garage. Here, the garage is your brain. We put all of our tools, sports equipment, and cleaning supplies (repeated activities) into tidy boxes (habits) and safely store them away in an easily accessible place so that we can use them when we need them. In doing this, we create plenty of space to park a shiny new car (something that needs brain power) in the garage where we can admire it, think about it and take care of it. Doing well in PA school is the shiny new car. You definitely need to create space for it and, believe me, that little beauty will require a big, clean, spacious garage to live in.

So how do you do this? Establish a routine and stick to it. Wake up at the same time each day and go to bed at the same time each night. Fall into a routine where you do the same thing every morning. For example, when you wake up in the morning, perhaps you will look over your schedule for the day and review your notes as you sip your coffee. Then you head out for a quick run, have some breakfast, make your lunch, clean up the kitchen, shower, brush your teeth, grab your gear for school and head out the door. Then, when you get back home, perhaps you will have a snack while you check your email, get dinner going, look over your notes from the day as you sit at the kitchen table, tidy up a bit, prepare the coffee maker for the morning, eat dinner, grab a cup of tea, go to your desk, study for a couple of hours, put everything you need for school the next day by the front door near your keys, brush your teeth, wash your face, lay out your clothes for the next day, put on your jammies and hop in bed.

Make sure that your routine incorporates ample time to study, as delineated by your schedule, and time for self-care. Make sure that you are occasionally scheduling in some stuff just for fun. The important thing in establishing a routine, whatever it may be, is that you do it day in and day out. You might need to tweak things here and there, but you will eventually find a rhythm that works for you.

If possible, automate what can be automated so that you can simply pay attention to what needs your attention (school). If you can, enroll in autopay for your bills. Doing so takes the hassle out of remembering to pay and frees up the time required to do it (I would recommend still looking over your bills, however, to make sure that everything is as it should be). Set up scheduled grocery deliveries and order household items from an online source. This eliminates the need to schlep over to the grocery store and can also help you stick to a budget because it decreases the likelihood of impulsive purchases. You can even take the guesswork out of your wardrobe by wearing very similar outfits each day. Hey, it worked for Steve Jobs!!

Ultimately, anything you can do to help you stay focused is beneficial. Remember that your time at PA school is a blip in time. Two or so years seems like a lifetime, but it goes by so quickly ... so, so very quickly.

Helpful hint: If you can attach a new habit to an established one, it is more likely to stick. Let's say that you sit down and drink a cup of coffee every morning. This is an established habit for you. It is something that you automatically do without much thought. Add the new habit of looking over your schedule and reviewing your notes to your old habit of sitting down and drinking coffee. After some time, you will automatically grab your schedule and notes as you automatically grab your cup of coffee.

Studying

What worked for you in undergrad will probably not work for you in PA school. There might be some trial and error in figuring out what does work and it might take you a while to find your footing, but don't worry; everyone else is in the same boat. You are on even playing field and everyone around you is pretty much feeling the same pressure to figure it all out. The goal in studying is to understand concepts and make connections. Cramming is never a good option.

Prepping For Lecture

Use your syllabus as a study guide because any and all objectives are fair game for testing, even if they are not thoroughly addressed in lecture. The syllabus contains all of the information about what is covered in which lecture and lets you know what reading materials, supplemental reading assignments and equipment may be necessary (for physical exam or diagnostic lab, for example).

Most programs use PowerPoint for lectures and some professors release their lectures a night or two before the lecture is scheduled. Take advantage of this and look over the lecture before class. Don't spend too much time here, though. You are not trying to retain information, but instead, simply becoming familiar with the content. You can also use this as an opportunity to make note of anything that is confusing or unclear.

Lecture

Now that you have prepared for lecture and have a decent sense of what will be covered, you can focus your attention on the material as it is being presented, actually listening and absorbing the material, rather than frantically trying to capture every word that the professor says as you type your notes. Try to take notes in your own words; rephrase things and make them your own. If, however, your professor has given a really great example or analogy that beautifully explains what is being taught or if the way that he or she says something really resonates with you, then writing verbatim makes sense.

Helpful hint: sometimes you need to crack open a book; sometimes you don't. Check with the second-year students to figure out which professors give you everything you need to know in the lecture and which ones expect you fill in the holes on your own. From there, you can decide how much time you should dedicate to reading the text.

A Word On Lectures

If your professor states something a couple of times or is very emphatic when saying something or, I don't know, says, "this is important", pay attention. That material will most likely make it onto the exam. Also, if you are in a modular program (a program where everything - from pathophys to pharm to physical exam – is presented in the context of a body system such as cardiology, pulmonology, dermatology, etc.) rather than in the more traditional model and you notice that the something is being said by multiple professors across multiple lectures, that's probably information that you should know.

After Lecture

Once lecture is over, you should review your notes as soon as possible, preferably on the same day. Again, most professors use PowerPoint and most students take notes in the "notes" section of the slides. It is easy to print the slides with your typed notes, or, if you prefer, you can create a Word doc from your notes. If you choose to create a document, it is a little easier to reorganize the information in a way that makes sense to you and, if you are searching for a keyword later, it is easy to find with Ctrl+F (which can be helpful for referencing during clinical year).

Once you have your notes organized, you have some options of how to proceed, which we will discuss in a moment. But first, word of caution: if you are someone who rewrites all of your notes over and over again, you need to find a new method of studying. The volume of material and the fast-paced curriculum are not amenable to this approach. You will fall behind.

Helpful hint: organization is key. You might find it helpful to create folders for each lecture on your laptop so that you can easily find them in the future (hint, hint ... this will come in handy for clinicals)

Study techniques

There are a couple of different approaches to studying. Again, it might be a process of trial and error but hopefully these recommendations will help you figure out what works best for you.

However you end up studying, the first step is to review your notes shortly after lecture and then reorganize them in a way that makes sense to you. Focus on the big picture. Once you have a firm grasp on the big concepts, you can move onto the more specific details.

Flashcards And Lists

Once you have everything organized, you have a couple of options of how to proceed next. You can make flashcards, lists and categories of lists, create diagrams and charts or use a combination of any or all of them. When I was in school, there were no Powerpoint lectures or laptops. Instead, professors used slide projectors and we were given handouts. The method that I used was to write notes in a separate notebook as I followed along with the handout during the lecture. Then, I would review my notes at some point that same day and make a list of all of the important information. I would fold my paper in half the long way and would write a question, statement, or definition on one side and then the answer on the other side. For example:

| - | Charcot's triad | - | Fever, jaundice, RUQ pain |
| - | Reynold's pentad | - | Above + AMS & low BP |

I used what I called the "cover-uncover" method, which pretty much consisted of me covering one side with an index card to see if I could get the right answer. Then I would go back through, this time covering the other side to see if I could get figure out what question, statement or definition was being referenced by the answer. I would go through this list a couple of times and if continued to get something wrong or felt that I didn't have a strong grasp of the material, I would highlight it, so that I would know to go back and study it again. My goal would be to do this within 24 hours of lecture. If at the end of the next round, I still got it wrong, I would put a red asterisk next to it. By this time, my list of red asterisked items would be kind of small, so I would write a new list and use that to continue to study. I would usually try to do this about three days after the material was first introduced. And finally, the night before the exam, I would again review everything, including the information that I understood in the first couple of rounds of studying. This is also a good time to fit in some group study, if that is your thing. In addition to the lists, I would make up patient vignettes that I would talk through either out loud to myself or with a study buddy.

Schedule recap:

Shortly after lecture (on the same day) – read lecture notes and make my list

Within 24 hours of lecture – go through the list a couple of times, highlighting items I needed to work on (round 1)

Within 72 hours of round 1 – go through the highlighted items and make my asterisked list (round 2)

Within another 24 hours or so of round 2 – go through the asterisked list (round 2)

A day or so before the exam – go through the entire list one more time; participate in a study group

Throughout the week or two leading up to the exam – create vignettes, talk through them, do any supplemental reading

This same technique can be used with flash cards. Any cards that contain information that you know well can be put to the side and cards that you need to keep working on will be put in a "tomorrow" pile. The next day, again within 24 hours, go back through the "tomorrow" pile. Put the cards that you need to work on into a new "tomorrow" pile and so on. Again, it is important to make sure that you go back and review the cards that you knew pretty well at the beginning of your study sessions. You want a comprehensive review before your exam. Then find a friend and quiz each other on the material. Maybe plan to do that the night before the exam.

Helpful hint: When you are studying, say everything out loud. Pretend that you are explaining whatever you are studying to someone else - be the professor talking to the class, be the provider explaining to the patient, be the preceptor explaining to the student. See how much you can say without looking at your notes and then go find a live person you can explain it to, whether it's your boyfriend, best friend, classmate, or the guy standing behind you in the deli line. If you can explain it, you understand it.

Pictures And Diagrams

For anatomy, physiology, and pathophysiology, drawing pictures and making diagrams and flowsheet can be helpful. What better way to learn the path of a red blood cell from the vena cava all the way to the aorta than by drawing a diagram of the heart and great vessels? Or if you are dissecting nerves and tracing their path in cadaver lab, what better way to become familiar with their expected courses and associated landmarks than drawing it out? And remember the coagulation cascade? You will once you make a diagram of it!

A helpful hint: if you use one of these techniques, you may consider purchasing some clear sheet protectors. Put your material into the sheet protectors and cover the answers on the actual paper with Washi tape. Write your answers on the sheet protector with a dry erase marker and then erase to start again. That way, you can quiz yourself over and over again until you feel super confident with the material.

Mnemonics And Acronyms

Mnemonics and acronyms, such as That Zebra Bit My Cookie (facial nerve branches – Temporal, Zygomatic, Buccal, Marginal mandibular, Cervical) and CRAB (multiple myeloma signs and symptoms – hyperCalcemia, Renal failure, Anemia, Bone pain), are helpful in remembering arteries, muscles and nerves in anatomy and also help with syndromes and constellations in clinical medicine.

Helpful hint: easily find tons of mnemonics and acronyms online. Just make sure that they make sense to you. If you can find a visual representation or create an outlandish story in your head about the mnemonic, you just might remember it more easily. For example, get crazy creative imaging a zebra biting your cookie. Fill in all the details of what kind of cookie he bit, what kind of facial expressions he made and how you felt when he bit your cookie. Sounds a little odd, but it works. If nothing else, you'll have a little fun while studying.

Charts And Tables

If you find that you need to compare and contrast information such as mechanisms of action, indications, contraindications or side effects of medications or you want to compare and contrast diseases such as asthma and emphysema, then charts and tables might be exactly what you need. Here again, the cover-uncover method will be helpful as you quiz yourself.

Patient Vignettes

In clinical medicine, we strive to learn who is at risk for what diseases (epidemiology), what causes certain diseases (etiology and pathophysiology), how diseases present (signs and symptoms), what tests we should order to diagnose diseases (diagnostics), how to treat and prevent diseases (treatment and prevention) and what the likely outcome of each disease is (prognosis and complications). We do this for each and every disease state that we learn about. If this seems like a lot of information, it is. If it seems kind of disjointed, it can be. But the best way to synthesize all of this information into cohesive understanding is to get a clear picture of what a patient with a certain disease looks like. You can start this process by creating charts and tables labeled with epidemiology, etiology, pathophys, signs/symptoms, diagnostic tests, treatment, complications, prevention, and prognosis and fill in the appropriate information. As you are getting comfortable with this information, you start to get an idea of what a typical patient with a particular disease looks like and acts like. Use this information to create scenarios, or vignettes, about that patient in which you ask and answer important questions.

Let's say that you are studying sickle cell disease. From your charts and tables, you know that a certain patient population is affected by sickle cell disease, that certain environmental conditions precipitate a sickle cell crisis, that there are common presenting symptoms, that there are potential complications associated with sickle cell disease and sickle cell crisis, that there are ways to treat and prevent crisis and that there are certain mortality and morbidity rates associated with the disease.

Now that you know all of this, ask yourself some questions and answer them in your vignette: "Mr. Troy is a 23-year-old African American male with ..... what is the best treatment? Why is that the best treatment? What complications is he at risk for developing? Why is he at risk for those particular complications? What patient education is most appropriate?" and so on. Honestly, I think that this is one of the highest yield methods that you can use (hint: remember when I suggested that you pay attention to something your professor says is important?). If you do this, the clinical picture of the disease state will come together for you. And guess what? That's the point. In fact, it is so important that faculty do pretty much the same thing when writing questions, or at least my colleagues and I did.

Study Groups

Study groups are great, as long as you are prepared. You must have good understanding of the material before you study in a group for a couple of reasons. First, you want to be able to contribute. If you are not prepared, you cannot contribute. Don't be that person. Secondly, and perhaps more importantly, studying with a group can shake your confidence if you do not have a decent handle on the material, especially when you compare your knowledge to that of the group members. I had an advisee who was very smart and capable, but she sabotaged herself by studying with a group when she wasn't quite ready to study with a group. Her BFF in class was part of the group, so she joined in because, you know, why not? Anyway, group study made her feel anxious and inadequate. She knew that this was not the best approach for her, but she was wanted to hang with her friends and was worried that her BFF would be upset if she broke off and studied on her own. Once she bombed a couple of tests, however, she knew that she had to switch up her studying style. But she was a little worried about what her BFF would think. You know what, though? Her BFF, who was also a wonderful, smart, lovely person totally understood and encouraged her to do what was best for her. Eventually, my advisee found her footing and was able to join that study group but timed it so that she used it as a review closer to the exam date, rather than a means to learn the material.

Some helpful hints about study groups:

Make sure that the group stays on task and on topic. Wandering happens.

Smaller groups of three or four work best.

Consider assigning topics of discussion for each group member.

Role play and act out scenarios. Make your vignettes come to life. Trust me, doing this leaves an impression and makes it easier to recall information at test time.

Studying with style

It might be worthwhile for you to identify whether you are an auditory, visual, or kinesthetic learner. Most people are a combination of all three, but one style usually predominates. There are tons of quizzes on the internet that can help you figure out your style if you don't already know what it is. Let's take a quick look what works best for each style.

Auditory Learner

Auditory learners learn best by, you guessed it, hearing information. So that means that listening in lecture is important. Get your hearing checked. If you are hearing impaired, see if accommodations can or need to be made.

Most lecturers use a microphone, but if you are having difficulty hearing what is being said, move closer to the front. Most programs record and post their lectures online and most of the sites to which they are posted allow you to listen to the recording at a higher speed, which makes review go more quickly. A word of caution, however, about recordings: sometimes they fail to record, sometimes the microphone doesn't work, sometimes the quality is poor and sometimes the site is down. Don't set yourself up for failure by relying on the recorded lectures as your primary source of information. Also, please do not record your professors unless you have clearly expressed permission to do so.

Read what you are studying out loud. When testing yourself with flashcards, say the words out loud.

Another great way for auditory learners to learn is to listen to podcasts. Of course, this is supplemental information, and it goes without saying that your primary source should be lecture materials, but you can easily listen to podcasts during downtime like when commuting, working out, making dinner, and doing household chores. You can do the same with videos, but just listen instead of watch. You could even record yourself as you are talking through questions and then listen again later.

Helpful hint: You know your ABCs, right? Singing the song in your head right now? Yeah, me, too. We remember information better when we put it to a melody. So, if you are struggling with remembering some information, make up a song about it!!

Visual Learner

If you are a visual learner, sit near the front of the class so that you can see everything clearly. Have your vision checked. If wear glasses, make sure that they are the correct prescription and make sure that the lenses are nice and clean. If you are visually impaired, check with you program to find out what accommodations can be made, if necessary.

Visual learners have the ability to close their eyes and recall what they saw in their mind's eye. So, the way that you organize your information is important. Using different colored pens for different concepts and highlighting, bolding, and underlining important concepts, ideas and information are good strategies. Also, charts, diagrams and tables are helpful, as are flashcards. Visual learners tend to remember how items are spatially related to one another on such study material. Post these things around your house so that you can glance at them as you go about your business. Watch supplemental videos.

Helpful hint: If you are listening to information, try to visualize what is being said.

Kinesthetic Learner

Kinesthetic learners need to move to process information, so sitting in lecture for four hours at a clip might be a challenge. Take breaks when you need to. Switch up the position you're sitting in. Ask if it would be ok if you stand in the back of the class for a little while. We had some students who would bring a bedside table that they adjusted to standing height in from the physical exam lab so that they could mix up standing and sitting during lecture.

While studying, walk around while you talk through a concept. Gesticulate, take up space, lay your flashcards out on the table to make a big game of memory out of them, get a large whiteboard that you can use to draw out diagrams and write down key information and concepts. Trace words with your fingers, chew gum, rock in a chair, tap your pen and bounce your foot while studying. Take frequent study breaks so you can get up and move around for a couple of minutes. Look at your notes while resting between sets when you're working out, have someone quiz you while you walk around campus and act out patient scenarios.

Study tips

Create A Study Schedule

Didactic year is pretty structured. For 8-12 hours per day, you are told where to go, whether it is sitting in lecture, working in the lab, taking assessments, or doing your volunteer work, and you are told what time to go there. More than likely, you will be provided with an electronic schedule that has blocks of time where you are expected to be somewhere doing one of those things. Whatever time is remaining is yours to schedule as you would like and I imagine that you would like to get some studying done during those times. The best way to approach studying is to schedule it and the best way to schedule it is to block off chunks of time on your calendar that you will dedicate to studying. Sit down at the beginning of the week and decide what you are going to study when. The hardest part is estimating just how much time you need to dedicate to studying. Try to distribute your workload fairly evenly throughout the week. Show up for your scheduled study the same way that you show up for class - on time and ready to go!

Interval Studying

One very important step in creating your study schedule is incorporating scheduled breaks. The Pomodoro method is an excellent example of a technique that does just that. In this technique, you set a timer for 25 minutes and go all in for active, distraction-free studying. This means that your phone is turned off, your browser is closed, your girlfriend has gone home, and you are focused in on learning. When the timer dings, you stop what you are doing and take a productive five-minute break. This combination of study time and break time is called a "chunk". Repeat this sequence for a total of four chunks, with the last chunk ending in a 15-minute break, rather than a 5-minute break. Then you can start the process over again.

What should you do during your break? Do something like go to the bathroom, stretch your legs and back, jog in place, take a couple of cleansing breaths, walk around, play with your dog, listen to music, have a healthy snack or step outside into the fresh air. When five minutes is up, it's time to get back to work.

None of this is set in stone, however. If you find that 25 minutes is too short or too long, make adjustments and do what works best for you. Personally, I like to work for 90 minutes and take 10-minute breaks for a total of 2 cycles. But you do you. You know what works best and if you don't yet, you'll figure it out.

If at any time during your study interval, you are nagged by a thought that just won't go away, write it down. For example, if you keep thinking how you can't forget to buy hot dogs for procedure lab, take a scrap piece of paper and write "buy hot dogs for procedure lab" on it so that you know that you won't forget it. By assuring yourself that you will remember to remember that nagging thought, you can let it go and get back to the task at hand.

Helpful hint: I know that screaming kids or barking dogs are sometimes unavoidable distractions. You may want to keep a pair of headphones or ear plugs handy, just in case you need to drown out any extraneous noise.

Give Your Body What It Needs

Make sure that you are well-hydrated, well-fed with nutritious foods and as well-rested as you can possibly be. Dehydration, sugar crash and all-nighters are not your friends here.

When To Study

There are different schools of thought on this one. Some say that the best time to study is early in the morning, while others believe that it is best to study is at the end of the day. Oh, what a luxurious concept: the thought of choosing this or that. You know that you'll be doing both, right?

Where To Study

You can study wherever you'd like as long as it is a quiet space where you can work uninterrupted. The temperature should be comfortable, you should have easy access to a bathroom, and you should be able to have some snacks and water handy. It should also be somewhere near your school or home (if it is not one of those places) so that you don't waste too much time travelling. In case you haven't noticed, time is a hot commodity in PA school. Shave a minute here, save a minute there. It all adds up!

What if I really, really, really don't want to study?

Procrastination happens, especially if you are tired, overwhelmed, don't like the material, or find the material too difficult. Ways to stave off that dreaded feeling are to eat well, stay hydrated, get adequate sleep, and embrace the process. If you are having difficulty understanding the material, ask a friend to explain it to you or go see your professor for help. If you have all of those ducks in a row, but are still fighting inertia, use the Two Minute Rule.

The Two Minute Rule states that you set a two-minute timer and work until the timer goes off. At the end of two minutes, commit to another two minutes. In most instances, just getting started is enough to get you going.

Taking exams

You will more than likely take your exam on your personal laptop using software that the school asked you to download. Make sure that you download the exam when you are supposed to download the exam. Don't wait until the last minute. Don't be the student who can't log in because you missed the window to download. Also, make sure that you have an up-to-date laptop that can handle the download. You don't want to be the person who has to run to IT during exam time because your computer crashed. You won't get that time back when you are finally able to start the exam. Don't make exam days harder than they have to be. They are stressful enough all on their own.

Most exams are multiple choice. That is because the Physician Assistant National Certifying Exam (PANCE) – you know, that exam you have to pass to become a PA-C - is multiple choice. Most programs model their question structure after the PANCE questions so that not only are you being tested but you are also practicing for taking the PANCE. Smart, right?

You will have straight-forward science questions, questions about how to interview, how to do a physical exam, diagnostic tests, and all sorts of other subject matter, but the bulk of what you will answer as you progress through the program will be patient vignettes and scenarios.

Hints For Multiple Choice Test-Taking

Read the questions carefully and pay attention to what is being asked. Sometimes the wording can be tricky. Sometimes answers are true statements, but they fail to adequately answer the question. Read each answer and choose the one that best answers the question.

Pay attention to key words such as pathognomonic signs or constellations of symptoms that are closely associated with a particular disease process. Be aware, however, that you may not see "malar rash", for example. Instead, there might be a description of what the rash looks like or there may be an accompanying photo.

Try to answer the questions without looking at the answers. If you get the right answer, you more than likely got the answer right.

Go through the test, answering questions that you know, skipping the questions that you don't know. Most exam software allows you to flag the questions so that you can come back to them later. Come back to your flagged questions and go through that process again. Sometimes info comes flying back into your head and sometimes another question reminds you of the answer.

Don't go back and change your answers. Your first answer is usually correct. Only change your original answer if you realize that you read the question incorrectly or that the answer you chose did not answer the question being asked. Otherwise, leave it alone. We had plenty of students who, when reviewing their exams, said, "I originally had the right answer, but I went back and changed it!!" Don't be that student.

The clinical medicine vignettes are designed to test your clinical knowledge and critical thinking skills. Don't read too much into them and don't add in your own details. Go with what is written in the question. Faculty are not trying to trick you.

Examine the answers and their relationship to one another. If there are two opposite answers, one of them is probably the right answer.

Answers with absolutes like "always" and "never" are not usually the right answer.

Pay particular attention to what you are being asked to answer in questions that contain words such as "even though", "although", "but", and "nonetheless".

Eliminate answers that you know are wrong. Some exam software allows you to put a line through an incorrect answer.

If you can narrow it down to two answers, you've got a 50/50 chance of getting it right. Ask yourself if one choice more completely answers the question more than the other. If you're still stuck, take turns imagining that each answer as the right answer, paying attention to how you feel as you imagine. I know this sounds kind of out there, but the answer that feels more wrong is probably wrong.

If "all of the above" and "none of the above" are answer options, they can be eliminated as correct if you know that one answer is wrong or one answer is correct, respectively.

If "all of the above" is an answer option and there are two answers that you know are correct, "all of the above" is likely the correct answer.

Helpful hint: getting good grades and performing well academically is great and gratifying and makes us feel smart and good and competent. But remember that the whole reason that we are going through all of this is to take care of real, live patients in the end. Real people with real problems and family and friends who love them. Huge responsibility. We strive to improve quality of life, save lives, make things better and to, above all else, do no harm. Being successful in didactic year isn't just so that we can pass exams and get good grades. The real reason that we want to do well is so that we can provide the very best, most competent patient care possible when we get to get out there and take care of patients.

Objective Structural Clinical Examination (OSCE)

What Is An Osce?

OSCEs are timed, simulated patient encounters. They are used to test your ability to elicit a patient history, whether focused or complete, perform an appropriate physical exam based upon the presenting problem and information obtained from the history, order and interpret diagnostic tests, create a reasonable differential diagnosis based upon all of the information gathered and then come up with a diagnosis and treatment plan, all of which you summarize in an oral presentation that you deliver to a proctor. Let's break this down a little more.

Chief Complaint

You will usually be provided with the chief complaint, patient demographics and the setting in which you are seeing the "patient" before you enter the exam. The chief complaint is the reason that the patient is coming to see you. An example: "Mrs. Smith is a 77-year-old African American female presenting to the primary care clinic with painful urination". This is a good time to start thinking about what might be causing her chief complaint.

History

You will most likely obtain the history from a faculty member or proctor who is acting as the patient and will respond to your questions from a script. Most programs will provide you with a rubric to use to prepare. The best way to study for eliciting a history is to actually elicit histories. Grab your rubric and practice with your classmates, family, and friends.

The patient's history includes the following:

Chief Complaint – you already know the chief complaint, but you should always ask the "patient" why he or she is coming to see you today.

History of Present Illness (HPI) – all of the details related to the problem. There are mnemonics to help you remember what to ask. One such mnemonic is OLD CART, which stands for onset (when did this start?), location (where is the symptom located?), duration (how long has this been going on?), characteristic (tell me more about the symptom. If, for example, the patient presents with pain, is it sharp, dull, lancinating, squeezing, throbbing, pressure, etc.), alleviating and aggravating factors/associated symptoms (what makes it better? What makes it worse? What other symptoms are you having?), radiation (does it go anywhere? Meaning, if there is pain in one area, does it stay there or move to another spot?), temporal relationship (does it come and go or is it constant?)

Review of Systems – this is a big laundry list of questions that span all of the body systems (constitutional, neurologic, cardiac, pulmonary, gastrointestinal, renal, hematologic, infectious, musculoskeletal, dermatologic, etc). Asking a review of systems list of questions helps you fill in any blanks that you missed in the HPI. Always ask about chest pain and shortness of breath, even if you are doing a history focused on something seemingly unrelated. You never want to miss a complaint of chest pain or shortness of breath. Also, unintentional weight loss is a big one because that symptom is often associated with an underlying malignancy.

Past Medical History – includes current and prior medical problems, vaccinations, hospitalizations, surgeries, and childhood illnesses

Medications – current medications, doses and schedule with any noted changes, additions, or discontinuations

Allergies – environmental, food and medication allergies

Social history – this includes occupation, living arrangements, how the patient tends to his or her activities of daily living (ADL's), whether or not the patient smokes, drinks or uses illicit drugs (or ever has), whether the patient exercises regularly, what kind of diet he or she eats and sexual history.

I know that this seems like a whole lot to remember, but don't be overwhelmed. The best way to remember all of this and to improve is to practice and you will practice this again and again and again.

Helpful hint: make sure that you verify patient identifiers (name, date of birth, medical record number) each step of the way, unless your program does not require that of you.

Physical Exam

You will perform physical exams on each other. Get comfortable with the idea of hanging out in a sports bra and shorts or just shorts, depending on your gender. For the OSCE, you will perform your physical exam under the observation of the proctor, who will give you a score based upon your technique, the completeness of the exam and the appropriateness of the selected physical examination maneuvers. In most programs, you are expected to verbalize what you are doing as you do it. There may be times when you are required to obtain vital signs and there will be times when they are given to you. Perform your exam bilaterally when applicable, unless told otherwise. Don't say "and I would do that on the other side, too". You must practice doing physical exams or you will fail. And you must practice doing physical exams while verbalizing what you are doing, or you will fail.

Make sure that you ask clarifying questions during your physical exam labs and ask for demonstrations if you are unsure of a technique.

Helpful hint: Just reading over the rubric is not adequate. Grab a timer, grab a friend, and get to examining. Practice verbalizing what you are doing as you are examining. Your goal is to get all of the components demonstrated with proficiency and complete the exam before time's up. You lose credit for whatever parts of the exam you don't get to before the timer goes off. Practice efficiency.

Diagnostic Testing

Depending on where you are in the didactic year, what is expected of you for this portion of the OSCEs will vary. When you are just starting out, you may be asked to simply state what tests you would order and why. As you progress through the program, though, you will be expected to interpret the results of what you order. Having a good understanding of what kind of information you get from each test is important. The most common diagnostic tests are the Complete Blood Count, Chem7, Comprehensive Metabolic Profile, Urinalysis and Chest X-ray. Know what they tell you and know when to order them.

Lab Tests

Remember that lab tests have a normal value range and that range can vary slightly from laboratory to laboratory and textbook to textbook. When you get a lab value, it usually comes with the normal range and is flagged, meaning emphasized in some way, to alert you of an abnormal result. Most programs will provide you will a normal range in testing situations. Of note, if the lab test result falls outside of that range, whether too high or too low, it warrants further investigation. Keep in mind that values that are too high and values that are too low mean different things and represent different types of disease processes. Here's a little more on some of the most common lab tests ordered:

Complete Blood Count (CBC) – If you want information about blood cell counts, this is your test. You can see the clue to that in the name. Most commonly, we look at the white blood cell count (WBC) to look for infection or evidence of blood cancers, the Hemoglobin and Hematocrit (H&H) to evaluate for anemia and the platelet count (plts) to get information about clotting ability. There are many more components to this test and there is a whole lot more information that can be gleaned from the results than what I just listed, but those are the most common.

If you are interested in metabolic function, Chem7 (sometimes called Basic Metabolic Profile – BMP), Chem10 and Comprehensive

Metabolic Profile (CMP) are the tests to order.

Chem7 – provides information about how the kidneys are working (BUN and creatinine), electrolyte balance (sodium, potassium, chloride, bicarbonate, or carbon dioxide) and blood glucose. Notice that there are 7 elements to the test.

Chem10 = Chem7 + extended electrolytes (magnesium, phosphorus, and calcium)

Comprehensive metabolic profile = Chem7 + liver function tests (total bilirubin, alanine aminotransferase, aspartate aminotransferase, alkaline phosphatase, albumin, total protein)

Anion Gap is an important element of the Chem7 or Chem10. It is a calculation that indirectly provides information about blood acidity. It is the value of the known cations (sodium + potassium) – the value of the known anions (chloride + bicarbonate). If the answer is outside of the normal range, it means that there are either some extra yet-to-be-discovered anions hanging around somewhere or that there is another acid-base imbalance that needs to be investigated further. FYI: most formulas calculate the anion gap without the potassium value (sodium – chloride + bicarbonate).

Imaging

The best way to become comfortable with interpreting imaging studies is to look at normal images over and over and over again. We learn by pattern recognition. The more normals you see, the easier it is to pick up on an abnormal. When reading images, pick an approach and use that same approach every time. Remember habits? With repetition, your chosen approach will become automatic, meaning that you will look at the imagines the same way each time without really needing to think about it. Why is this important? Because you won't have to waste time thinking about what to do and, more importantly, if you consistently do something the same way each time, you are much less likely to miss something. Honestly, if you can't find what you are looking for, what's the point of ordering the test in the first place?

For example, when reading chest x-rays, you can use ABCDEFGH, which stands for tracheA, Bones, Cardia, Diaphragm, Effusions, lung Fields, Gastric bubble, Hilum. With this approach, you first look at the trachea (a reminder to look at the airways), then move onto the bones (all of them), then the heart, the diaphragm, the costovertebral angles (this is where the effusions would be found), stomach (gastric bubble) and the structures in the middle of the chest (hilum). I know that this probably seems more confusing than helpful at this point, but keep this section in mind and refer back to it when you start learning about how to read imaging. It will make much more sense.

Here's the most important thing about ordering diagnostic tests: you have to look at the results. If you don't follow up the results, you might as well not have ordered anything in the first place.

Helpful hint: if your patient has old lab values and imaging available, please make sure that you look at them and compare them with the labs or imaging you have in front of you. Patients with chronic disease can have different baseline normal labs and so an abnormal finding on current labs may, in and of itself, be an abnormal finding, but might be normal for that patient. A good example is chronic kidney disease. Patients with chronic kidney disease have higher BUN and creatinine levels at baseline, meaning that these numbers are higher for them, even when they are not sick. Comparing current lab values to old lab values lets you know a couple of things. First, you can determine what IS normal for the patient and secondly, you can compare your new lab findings to the old (normal for that patient) findings to see if the new findings are normal for that particular patient.

Oral Presentation

The oral presentation is your opportunity to present your findings and discuss what you think is going on with the patient, based upon those findings. Generally, you start with the patient demographics and the reason that the patient came to see you. Then you relate the pertinent HPI findings, being sure to include all of the relevant positive and negative review of system answers, as well as social history, medical history, medications and allergies. Then move onto your physical exam findings, including vital signs. Again, make sure to include any normal and abnormal findings that are pertinent to the presenting problem (this will make more sense as you start to do physical exams). Next, you discuss your differential diagnosis (more on that in a minute), why you picked what is in your differential and what you think is the most likely diagnosis. Once you state your most likely diagnosis, you discuss your treatment plan including any medications, further testing, referrals or consultations, patient counseling and disposition (where the patient will receive said treatment – in the hospital, at home, in a nursing home, etc.).

In most instances, you will receive a rubric or instructions on what is expected from you when you do your oral presentation. You will present your patient to a proctor, usually a faculty member, who will score your presentation. Again, the best way to do well in oral presentations is to practice presenting orally. Grab your rubric and get to work. It is helpful to study with a classmate because you may find that you like his style or adopt the way that he phrases stuff. Or you might just be that inspiration for someone else.

Helpful hint: your job as the presenter is to lead the listener to your conclusion. Oral presentations are generally expected to be presented as outlined above. Try really had to stick to that order (patient demographics, chief complaint, hpi, physical exam, etc.). When information is presented out of order, it is confusing for the listener and makes it harder to follow your train of thought.

Differential Diagnosis

A differential diagnosis is a list of potential causes of your patient's symptoms. I like to think of it as focused, organized brainstorming. Generating a differential diagnosis is important because if you don't think of something, you can miss is. There are many different approaches to generating a differential and there are tons of mnemonics used to help you make sure that your differential is broad, meaning that it includes lots of different possibilities. There are even apps and tools out there. When you hear a chief complaint, you should start to generate a differential. Your differential will then guide you on what kind of questions to ask, what components of the physical exam are important and what tests you will order to rule in or rule out the items on your list.

Let's say that a patient presents with chest pain. Take second right now to look up "chest pain differential diagnosis". The possibilities seem endless, right? That's because chest pain is a complaint that generates a wide differential because anything in the chest (skin, muscles, nerves, blood vessels, lungs, heart, bones) can cause pain and anything near the chest can cause referred chest pain (stomach, gallbladder, pancreas, liver, diaphragm). There are also psychological causes of chest pain, although psychological causes of somatic complaints are diagnoses of exclusion, meaning that you usually rule out any physical causes before you begin to entertain a psychologic reason.

Now that you have a differential in mind, you can narrow it down by asking questions. Certain disease processes are associated with certain symptoms, physical exam findings and diagnostic results. Also, patient demographics and past medical history are important when generating a differential. For example, a healthy child who has chest pain is very unlikely to have pain due to a heart attack. The child has different "most likely" reasons for chest pain than an elderly person.

Let's use chest pain as an example. When we hear chest pain, one of the things we think about is acute coronary syndrome. We think of that because we know that acute coronary syndrome can be deadly if missed and we certainly don't want to miss anything that can kill our patients. That being said, although we think of acute coronary syndrome, it is not the only thing on our differential because not everyone who has chest pain has acute coronary syndrome. Hence, the wide differential.

So, now that we have this wide differential, how do we figure out what is or is not on the "most likely" (aka differential diagnosis) list? We ask questions. We ask questions from OLD CART and from our review of systems. The answers to those questions lead us toward or away from diagnoses. Acute coronary syndrome is less likely if, for example, upon questioning, you learn that the pain is unilateral, burning in nature and located in a dermatomal distribution. Asking about location and quality of pain is built into OLD CART (kind of smart, no?). Because you are a very good student, you generated a wide differential and, because your differential was wide, you had herpes zoster on your list. Guess what? Unilateral, burning pain in a dermatomal distribution is *very* characteristic of herpes zoster. Not so much so for acute coronary syndrome. Acute coronary syndrome, therefore, moves down on your list of differentials to less likely and herpes zoster moves up as most likely. Then you do your physical exam, making sure to look for the presence or absence of pertinent exam findings. Whether or not certain exam findings are present on or absent on examination helps you to further prioritize your list of differentials. If you find a vesicular rash atop an erythematous base that is in a dermatomal distribution that does not cross midline, then you pretty much have your diagnosis of herpes zoster.

If, however, your patient presents with crushing substernal chest pain with radiation to the left arm, neck, and jaw in association with nausea, diaphoresis, and a sense of impending doom, then this is not herpes zoster. There is something much more ominous going on here. Makes sense?

In some instances, all you need to make your diagnosis is information obtained from your history and physical. Herpes zoster is one such diagnosis. Sure, you could send off a sample of the vesicular fluid for testing, but doing so is not necessary for diagnosis. Other times, however, we need diagnostic tests to help us figure out what is going on. The patient with substernal, crushing chest pain needs more work up and needs it quickly because his symptoms point to something potentially deadly like acute coronary syndrome. In such cases, the diagnostic data is helpful to rule in or rule out suspected disease processes (he has acute coronary syndrome or he does not). The next best step in the care of the patient is usually based on what is revealed in that testing and the overall picture of the patient.

The point here is that generating a differential diagnosis allows you to think of things that you might not have thought about, which makes it harder to miss something.

Helpful hint: If you are in a modular program, whatever system you are in is the one being tested. For example, the source of chest pain will not be herpes zoster if you are in your cardiology module. Faculty are not trying to trick you (hint: look at your rubric).

Physical exam lab

Physical exam lab is where you practice the physical exam maneuvers that you learn. There will usually be a professor or two hanging out to demonstrate techniques, answer your questions and provide feedback on your skills. You will practice all aspects of the physical exam, from taking vital signs to examining the skin to listening to heart sounds to testing muscle strength and everything in between, on each other. You will take turns being the examiner and the examined.

 The exception to this is what we call the "sensitive exams", meaning genital, rectal and breast exams. These particular exams will be practiced on a mannequin or in many cases, PA programs send their students to a facility, usually a medical school, where live models, who give real-time feedback as you are examining them, help you learn how to properly perform these exams. The idea of this is usually quite anxiety-inducing for PA students due to the sensitive nature of the exams and because these exams are typically the first time that students are performing a 'real' exam on a real person who is not their classmate or family member. This reaction is perfectly normal. Rest assured, however, that the experience is well worth it. And it is not as bad as you imagine it to be. As soon as you start examining, all of those nerves fade away and you realize what an incredible learning opportunity you have been afforded. Plus, once you get out there in clinical rotations, that first exam on your first patient will be a piece of cake.

Procedures lab

Procedures lab presents an opportunity for you to practice doing procedures such as IV insertion, phlebotomy, bladder catheterization, nasogastric tube insertion, lumbar puncture, punch biopsy, suturing, etc. Some programs allow you to practice simple procedures such as phlebotomy on each other, while in other programs, all of your procedures are done on a dummy. When I was in school, we drew each other's blood and practiced inserting nasogastric tubes on each other. That was quite an experience, but in my opinion, well worth it. Obviously, more invasive procedures such as lumbar punctures and intubations are not something that you will be practicing on your classmate.

Use the rubric and text to prepare beforehand and watch some videos demonstrating technique. Coming in prepared makes the lab more rewarding because you are actually practicing, rather than trying to catch up on what you should have already learned.

Some programs will allow you to visit the lab after hours, while others will not, so it is important to get in all the practice you need during scheduled lab time. This is especially true if the procedure involves using something that is a potential liability for the school, such as sharps, for example.

Make sure that you are dressed appropriately and have all the necessary equipment. If you were supposed to buy hotdogs to practice punch biopsies, make sure that you do that.

Helpful hint: if you cannot physically practice a procedure or skill, visualize yourself doing it. See yourself going through all of the steps in your head. Visualization lights up the same neural pathways as physical practice.

Cadaver lab

I'm not going to lie. I kind of hated cadaver lab. Our lab was on Wednesday mornings and every single Wednesday morning right through to the last Wednesday morning, I had I would call "GI distress". Let's just leave it at that. But it wasn't necessarily the dead bodies that bothered me. I had seen dead bodies before when I worked as an emergency room. As an ER tech, I would help the nurses clean and prepare the body for viewing by family. Of course, there was a certain sadness to this and seeing families say goodbye to their loved ones was heartbreaking, but it was also a very meaningful task. I felt like taking care of the body was one last respectful gesture, one last act of kindness that we could do for the patient and, by extension, for the family. As a student in cadaver lab, though, I felt intrusive. The idea of dissecting a person was very off-putting to me, even though I understood the purpose and was grateful for the opportunity. What got me through, though, was knowing that we were honoring the wishes of the people who so generously donated their bodies so that we could learn from them. If you think about it, it's a really special person who makes such a selfless contribution.

Our cadavers were fresh, meaning that they had not been dissected yet. This may or may not be the case for you because bodies are in short supply. Having the opportunity to work on a fresh body was, from an education point of view, amazing because we were able to dissect everything ourselves. No one else had been there yet. But, from an emotional point of view, working on a fresh body was harder because we had to make the first cuts. I will admit that seeing our bodies' hands and faces were probably the hardest parts to see. Our lab kept the faces covered until we were ready to work on that area of the body.

You will work on your body as a group. Find your balance with your group. If you love to dissect, have at it! If not, do something else helpful like help find landmarks, have the dissection book at the ready or hand tools to your partner who is elbow deep in a body cavity. There are plenty of ways to contribute and learn.

The lab itself is cold. This is a good thing, even for those of us who are perpetually cold. That is because you will more than likely be wearing some sort of protective plastic gown or apron, mask, goggles, and gloves, all which make you hot. And, if you are anything like me, nervousness combined with a hot room is a surefire recipe for wooziness.

Speaking of wooziness, make sure that you put something in your belly before lab. I'm not talking bacon, eggs, and a side of home fries, but something light that will keep your stomach settled. Try not to lock your knees while standing and flex your calves and thighs every now and then to keep your blood circulating. If you do start to feel pass out-y, step away, go sit down somewhere (preferably outside of the lab) and put your head between your knees. Have something to drink and get back in there when you feel steadier.

The worst part of cadaver lab is the smell and the slippery floors (all of that preservative fluid has to go somewhere once you start making cuts). Make sure that you wear non-slip shoes and old clothes that you wear only in cadaver lab (bring a change of clothes). You don't want to slip and fall into whatever is on the floor and you don't want to smell like cadaver lab outside of cadaver lab. Also, clean your instruments well. You don't want to bring pieces of cadaver lab home with you.

Formaldehyde smells terrible and it seems to linger in your nose far beyond the end of lab. Some say that you get used to the smell.

I did not. If you start to feel overwhelmed, step outside. I've heard that putting lavender oil or tea tree oil into your mask helps, although I've never tried that.

Helpful hint: Do not wear skirts, flip flops, shorts or any other clothing that will leave your skin exposed. Splashes happen. Pieces fall off of the table onto your foot.

Faculty

Here's what surprised me the most about being a faculty member: the lengths that faculty go to to help you succeed. Every step of the program is thoughtfully and painstakingly planned out and re-evaluated and reworked, when necessary. Nothing is haphazard or extraneous; everything that is in the curriculum serves a specific, well thought out purpose. Because faculty have high standards and expectations for the profession, they have high standards and expectations from you, the student, and from each other, as those responsible for educating you, the up-and-coming PA's. This means that the academics are rigorous and the code of conduct is strict. Your job, as the student, is to rise to the challenges of PA school with maturity, motivation, diligence, and grace. If you are struggling, please reach out early on. The earlier that faculty can intervene, the better your chances of successfully overcoming whatever it is that you are struggling with. They are pulling for you and are so very proud when you make it across that graduation stage. Trust me, I know.

My goal in PA school was to put my head down, learn lots of stuff and stay under the radar. Here are some helpful hints to keep you under the radar:

There will be times when you are angry, frustrated and upset about what a faculty member does or says, you might not like the policies or schedule, you might think that mandatory volunteer hours are stupid, and you might find that you thoroughly dislike a particular professor. That's ok. We feel how we feel. Be sure to conduct yourself, however, with professionalism. Be careful with your words and actions. PA school is a small community. Things get back to professors.

Be sure to be respectful in your interactions with faculty, staff, and each other. Behavior is noticed.

Be settled and ready to go before your professor walks in the room. Walking in on time is late.

Be prepared and ready to participate. No professor likes standing at the podium, asking what she feels is a simple question and getting crickets for a response.

Lecture can be boring. Honestly, I bored myself sometimes when I was up there teaching. Try not to talk or be disruptive.

You will need letters of recommendation at some point, right?

What if I'm failing?

If you are failing or teetering on the edge of failure, seek out help early. Professors like the proactive, self-aware student. Faculty will only reach out if they notice something is wrong and they usually don't notice that something is wrong until you fail an assessment. By that point, you have probably been struggling for a while and are in pretty deep. Be an advocate for yourself and make all efforts to stay ahead of that. Your advisor is always a good place to start.

Be familiar with the remediation process and do all of the work required of you in that process, should you find yourself there. Your student handbook is a good resource here, as is your advisor.

CLINICAL YEAR

As didactic year comes to a close, you will find yourself feeling feelings that are similar to the feelings you felt at the start of school. Some may feel super excited, completely confident, and ready to go, while others may be plagued with nervousness, self-doubt and perhaps even a sense of dread. I remember the day that I started my first clinical. I felt like I was going to throw up because I was so nervous. I was worried that I wasn't good enough or smart enough. I was worried that I would make a fool of myself, that I would stammer when I talked or that I would get lost in the bowels of the hospital, never to be seen again. I worried that patients would kick me out of their rooms, demanding to see someone more competent. But, guess what? Once I got there, I did fine. In fact, I did better than fine. I did great. And I loved it. I loved seeing patients. I loved applying what I had learned. I loved that the right answers sometimes just came flying out of my mouth, surprising myself with my knowledge. Did I still feel insecure sometimes? Of course.

Did I feel overwhelmed at times? No doubt.

Did I feel inadequate every now and them? Yup.

Were my presentations always stellar? Nope.

Did the occasional patient refuse to be seen by a student? Yes.

But did I feel unprepared? No way. And neither will you. Trust me, you are more prepared than you think you are and you know much more than you think you do.

What to expect

In most cases, you will get your clinical year schedule at the end of didactic year. Your program will facilitate the onboarding process for each of your sites at that time, as well.

Core rotations include Inpatient Internal Medicine, Outpatient Medicine/Family Medicine/Primary Care, Women's Health, Pediatrics, General Surgery, Psychiatry and Emergency Medicine. Depending on the program, rotations last anywhere from four to eight weeks. Some programs offer one to two elective rotations, which can be an additional couple of weeks spent at one of the core rotations or can be time spent with specialty disciplines such as Plastic Surgery or Gynecology Oncology, for example. Some programs allow you to set up your own rotations. If, for example, you want to do your internal med rotation at the hospital in your hometown, your program might let you coordinate that, as long as the site meets the rotation requirements.

Potential preceptors include attending physicians, resident physicians, physician assistants and nurse practitioners. You may work one on one with a provider, or you may be a part of a team that includes other PA students and/or medical students. It all depends upon the structure and culture at your assigned site.

Your program will inform you of what is expected of you while on rotations and will let you know how your performance will be assessed, usually in the form of end-of-rotation exams and preceptor evaluations. Additionally, you will find out how the program will support you while you are out there in the clinical world. Usually, everything goes as expected, but should you find yourself in a situation where you need further guidance or assistance, the protocol for that should be clearly delineated for you.

Before your rotation

Look to your clinical year director for guidance on when and how to contact your preceptor. Usually, it is advisable to reach out to the contact person at least one to two weeks prior to the start of your rotation to find out where you should go, where you should park, whether you need to stop by security for badges or parking passes and what you should wear (scrubs or professional versus business casual attire).

If you can, take a drive to your clinical site before your rotation begins. Map out the route and figure out how long it takes to get there, being mindful that if you are going to be driving during rush hour, you will probably need to add a couple more minutes onto your travel time. When you arrive, see if you can find where you will be parking and then see how long it takes you to get from your car to the building, office, or department where your clinical is being held. Sometimes it is simply a matter of walking across the parking lot, other times it is a walk around the block, through a couple of buildings and up a couple of floors.

Gather all of the materials that you will carry around with you and make sure that your white coat is clean and wrinkle-free.

Helpful Hint: just because your white coat has four pockets, it doesn't mean you have to fill them all. You should definitely bring your stethoscope, a pen, a little pad to write on, a small reference book, pen light, reflex hammer, Snellen chart, a healthy, portable snack and a couple of bucks. Anything beyond that, unless recommended by the site, is extraneous. Ask ahead of time if you can carry your phone with you. Some places are touchy about that. And if you do carry your phone with you, keep it put away.

On Rotation

Professionalism

Be respectful in your appearance, attitude, and interactions. Not just because it's the right thing to do, but also because you represent your program at the clinical site and sites are hard to procure. You know what that that means? That means that you will be in deep doo-doo if you do something on rotation that makes them think twice about accepting students from your program in the future. Behave in a way that would make your program proud. In fact, behave in a way would make your mom, dad, grandma, sister, auntie, second cousin and kindergarten teacher proud.

Come Early And Stay Late

Be on time and by "on time", I mean five minutes early. Don't be the person scurrying up, all out of breath and sweaty, to your preceptor just as the clock strikes the time you are due to arrive. And don't be late. Nobody is interested in your excuses for tardiness. Demonstrate through your actions that you respect your preceptor's time and are appreciative of his or her willingness to share their wisdom, insight, and experience. Whether you realize it or not, precepting is difficult. It is a huge time commitment and a potential liability. But usually those who agree to precept love to precept and that's a really good thing.

Stay until all of your work is done and make sure that you have followed up on all of the stuff that you were supposed to follow up on. Make sure to ask if there is anything else you can help with before you go. Do not leave without first getting the OK from your preceptor, even if you are leaving later than your scheduled time to leave.

Know Your Role

It is important to know your role and to know what behavior and interactions are appropriate for you as a student. Your preceptor will decide when and how you interact with your patients and most will need to get a sense of who you are before they let you loose in their department. This is especially true in the operating room. If you demonstrate that you can properly scrub in (and yes, you must demonstrate that you can do that before you can step foot inside), you will be allowed to stand in the OR. From there, you may be invited to step closer and hold a retractor. Be interested. If you are not interested, at least act interested. Ask meaningful questions and listen to the answers. The person sharing his or her wisdom and insight is clearly invested in the subject and in sharing his or her knowledge with you. Show them the courtesy of interest. Do not be annoyed that you are not doing as much as you think you should be doing. It is true that this is your educational experience, but what supersedes the importance of that is the care of the patient and if, for whatever reason, your preceptor thinks it is best that you stand and observe, then you stand and observe.

Same goes for procedures. Typically, procedures are taught in a "see one, do one, teach one" manner, which means that you will probably observe a procedure a time or two before you are able to actually get to get in there and get your hands dirty (figuratively, of course. You will be wearing gloves). If you are simply observing, be grateful that you are observing and make the best of it. Be proactive: offer to help set up or clean up, volunteer to grab supplies, hold the patient's hand for reassurance, ask questions. Sometimes you won't be asked to participate. That's just the way it is.

Basically, be prepared to observe patiently, be patient while being observed and follow your preceptor's lead. You may start off just shadowing, but you will eventually be allowed to see the patients on your own and then report back to the preceptor. When they think you are ready, they will let you know. Of course, if you are halfway through your rotation and you are still just shadowing, then there is a problem, either with your preceptor or with their perception of you. If you find yourself in a similar situation, reach out to your program for guidance.

Conversely, you should never be asked to do something that you are unqualified to do and you should never do something that you are unprepared to do. Don't be afraid to say that you are uncomfortable doing something that you really shouldn't be doing anyway.

Basically, you are the low man on the totem pole. You will not be the one swooping in to perform emergency tracheostomies or whisking patients away for other life-saving interventions. But, you might have the privilege of witnessing some really interesting cases, which makes for great stories to share at call-back.

Communication

As we all know, the two components of communication are talking and listening. As you recall, the way that we communicate our patients' information to the preceptor is in the oral presentation. You should, at this point in your PA student career, be able to give a concise recap of the patient's history of present illness including all pertinent positive and negative review of system questions and appropriate physical exam findings, including what you did and did not find that will support your most likely diagnosis. You should be able to generate a simple differential and tell the preceptor what you think the next best step is. Your preceptor may not agree with your assessment and plan and that is ok. This is a great opportunity to learn. You are not expected to function as a full-fledged provider. You are there to learn, so take the opportunity to learn. Embrace this process. Be open to constructive criticism. Ask questions to help develop your critical thinking skills and make sure that you incorporate what you learn from that into your future interactions.

Honestly answer any questions asked of you. If your preceptor asks if the patient smokes cigarettes and you forgot to elicit a social history, admit it. If you didn't check for CVA tenderness and you really should have, admit it. Then offer to go back and do what you forgot to do. Don't document a physical exam finding if you didn't physically examine the patient and don't put words into your patients mouth in an attempt to save face. Don't make stuff up. Nobody likes a liar.

If your preceptor asks you what the best test is to rule out a pulmonary embolism or why a patient with chronic kidney disease should not use ibuprofen, and you don't know the answer, your response should be something like "I'm not sure, but I'll look it up and get back to you". Then go look it up and get back to her. Never answer with "I don't know" and leave it at that. It makes you seem uninterested, unmotivated, and lazy.

Helpful hint: asking questions is an important part of the learning process. Make sure, though, that the questions you ask are not ones that you can easily answer on your own… you know, simple stuff you can easily look up.

Nurses

Make friends with the nurses. They can make or break you. They can make you look brilliant or make you feel incompetent. They can teach you tips and tricks that you can't learn from anyone else. Let them teach you how to insert IV's, troubleshoot Dobhoff tubes and place foley catheters (if, of course, you are credentialed to do that – check with your preceptor first). They are a wealth of knowledge and an integral part of the healthcare team. They know their patients like no one else, so if you want the down-low, talk to the nurses.

While on inpatient rotations, your day shift will start by finding out what happened with your patients overnight. Even if there is an overnight provider who gives you sign-out about your patient's overnight events, always talk with the nurse, as well. He or she will likely have more insight about the patient and can tell you more details about overnight events. Make sure that you ask if he or she has any concerns that they want you to bring up on rounds that day. We should make it as easy as possible for nursing staff to have their concerns heard and addressed.

Writing Notes

During didactic year you will learn about all of the different types of notes that you will need to know how to write and you will receive instruction on the format, content, and purpose of each note. This is because we do a whole lot of written communication in medicine. By the time you get to clinicals, you will have written a ton of notes in your history-taking class. Here is a brief introduction to some of the more common notes.

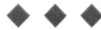

History and Physical

This is the note that is written when a patient is admitted to the hospital. It starts with the chief complaint and then progresses through the HPI, physical exam findings, laboratory data, assessment of the patient and your plan for each problem. Somewhere in there (style dictates where) is the emergency department (ED) course, meaning a summary of what happened while they were in the ED and what was done for the patient while they were in the ED. If a patient is a direct admission (directly admitted to the floor without going through the emergency department), then there obviously is no ED course. Once all of that information is documented, you create an assessment and a plan. The assessment summarizes what you think is going on with the patient and the plan is an outline of how you are going to take care of the patient. There are generally two ways to list the problems. One is "by problem" and the other is "by system". Let's say that someone is being admitted with gastroenteritis, dehydration, and acute kidney injury. Here is how each set of problems would be addressed with "by plan" and "by system".

"By plan":

1. Problem #1 (gastroenteritis)-- Plan #1
2. Problem #2 (dehydration) – Plan #2
3. Problem #3 (acute kidney injury) – Plan #3

"By system":

Neuro –

Cardiovascular –

Respiratory –

GI – gastroenteritis: plan #1

GU – dehydration: plan #2, acute kidney injury: plan #3

Endo –

Heme/Onc -

ID -

For the blanks in the "by systems" list, you can either write "no active problems" or you can list normal findings. For example, "alert and oriented" under Neuro, "heart rate and blood pressure withing normal limits" under Cardiovascular and "satting well on room air, nothing acute on chest x-ray" under Respiratory, and so on. Both are equally sufficient. Look to your preceptor to decide which style you use.

SOAP note

The SOAP note is used for problem-focused visits and for progress notes. Problem-focused visits are visits in which you focus on the problem that brings the patient in to see you. Sore throat, headache, constipation, etc. The SOAP note is also used in the inpatient setting as a progress note. A progress note is the note used to document the patient's hospital stay on a day-to-day basis.

S – subjective. What the patient has to say (an abbreviated HPI essentially)

O – objective. Objective findings. Physical exam findings, laboratory data.

A – assessment. What you think is going on.

P – plan. How you will address what is going on.

Progress notes usually start with a section called "overnight events". In this section, you state what happened overnight. If nothing of significance happened, "nothing overnight" is sufficient. If something did happen, describe what happened ("received 5mg of IV haldoperidol for agitation with good effect", for example).

Discharge Summary

Discharge summary is a note that is written when the patient is ready to leave the hospital. This note usually summarizes why the patient came to the hospital, why she was admitted, what happened during her admission and what makes her ready to be discharged. This note should include documentation of the physical exam findings upon discharge, laboratory data upon discharge, a list of home medications, a list of medications upon discharge, rationale as to why any home medications were stopped or changed and why and new medications were added, patient disposition (where is the patient is going to go: home, home with services, nursing home, rehab facility, etc.) and discharge instructions for the patient, including suggested follow up appointments. A copy of the discharge summary should be sent to any receiving facility, the patient's primary care provider and any consultants who will see the patient in follow-up.

Inpatient Rounds

On your internal medicine and surgery rotations you will see the same patients for days in a row. It is your job to know absolutely everything about your patient. If your attending or preceptor asks a question about your patient, you should easily be able to answer it. If not, you should be able and willing to quickly find out. Know their social history, know their home meds with doses and schedules, know their medical history and know everything about their current and most recent past hospitalizations. If your attending wants to know how many cycles of chemotherapy your patient underwent twenty years ago for treatment of his cancer, find out and do it quickly. As a student, you will carry a smaller patient load than the other members of the team. You should know your patients in and out.

Ask thoughtful questions, but not too many. You want to be inquisitive and engaged, but not disruptive and pesky. If your attending is bestowing nuggets of wisdom, make sure that you write them down so you remember them for next time. Attendings don't like to answer the same questions again and again.

On rounds you discuss your patients with your care team, which is usually comprised of an attending physician and any combination of the following: residents, physician assistants, nurse practitioners, the nurses caring for the patients and other students. The first step in preparing for rounds is to find out about any overnight events and to review their charts for vital signs and laboratory data. Review the note from the day before to make sure that you are aware of any existing problems and to see what goals were set by the team for the patient and whether or not they were met. Then go see your patient. Ask them how they are doing and ask specific questions about their existing problems. If, for example, a patient was admitted with pancreatitis, ask him how his pain is. After you have gathered all of your data, go write your note. You will use your note to present your patient to your team.

Speaking of goals, your attending and/or preceptor will give you things to do, based upon what is going on with the patient: "Check a CBC in the afternoon", "consult cardiology", "get a stat head CT", "calculate the FeNa", "get her records from that other hospital". Make sure that you do what is asked of you and make sure that you follow up on what you do. Find out the CBC result, read the cardiology consult note, order that stat head CT and find out the results, calculate the FeNa and get those hospital records. If you aren't sure how to do what is asked of you, touch base with your preceptor. If you were unable to do what was asked of you, you better have a good reason why. When you get results, tell your preceptor what you think and what you'd like to do about them. Do not do things without checking in with your preceptor, unless, of course, he or she has given you clear instructions to do otherwise.

Some tips:

Present you patients in the same way that the group does. Most usually start with overnight events. Make sure that you follow convention.

Make sure that anything abnormal (vital sign, lab value, physical exam finding) is addressed in your note.

Document what lines (peripheral IV lines, central lines, tunneled catheters, PICC lines, chest tube, drains, NT tubes, foley catheters, etc.) the patient has, how long they have had them, whether or not they still need them and what the 24-hour output was for lines that put stuff out (foleys, chest tubes, drains, NG tubes)

If your patient is on antibiotics, document what day out of how long the treatment will last (day 2/5, for example)

If you are on a surgical service, it is important to document what post-operative day it is for the patient, as well as whether the patient is passing gas, having bowel movements, or taking a diet. Surgeons love to hear about that stuff.

Also, not the state of the incision site. Clean, dry, and intact is what you're aiming for.

If the patient has as-needed medications ordered, it is always good to know how much he or she required in the past 24 hours.

Document if your patient is in restraints, noting what kind of restraints are being used, and laterality (right soft holder wrist, bilateral untied mitts, locked 4-point, etc.) and why they are still necessary.

Document any drips, current doses and whether those doses have changed (norepinephrine 10mcg/min, normal saline 75ml/hr, etc.)

Documentation of urine output and total intake and output balance is important, especially if someone is hemodynamically unstable or has heart, liver, or kidney failure.

Seeing Patients

Always introduce yourself to patients and their families and always tell them that you are a PA student. Transparency is important. When you see a patient, you enter into an unspoken contract. The patient agrees to be seen by you and you agree to do your best to take good care of him or her to the best of your ability. Above all else, honor this contract. Do not make promises or assertions that you have no authority to make and if you do not know the answer to a question that a patient or family asks, be honest and tell them that you do not know, but you will discuss it with your preceptor. Don't let arrogance or fear cloud your judgement. If you don't know what you are doing or are unclear about what you are supposed to do, ask for help. If your preceptor told you to do something and you didn't really understand the instructions, ask for clarity. Don't put your patient's care in jeopardy because you don't want to look stupid. Here is one of the most important qualities of a good physician assistant: know what you know and know what you don't know. Medicine is a huge, ever-growing, ever-evolving discipline. It is impossible for anyone, especially a student, to know everything. It is your job to ask for help, even if it means calling the condescending, borderline abusive consultant at 3:00 am to ask for guidance. Do what is in the best interest of the patient. Ask yourself, "what would I do if this was my Grandma" (or anyone else you love dearly) and treat your patient in the manner that you would want your loved one to be treated. Go the extra mile and do the right thing.

When talking with patients, avoid medical jargon. Think again about Grandma. Would she understand "well, ma'am, you are having trouble breathing because you have florid pulmonary edema secondary to your longstanding hypertensive heart disease and subsequent low ejection fraction which results in a decreased ability of your body to meet its metabolic demands"? Or would something like "your heart is like a pump that pushes your blood forward to the rest of your body. Because you have had high blood pressure for so long, your heart doesn't work in quite the same way that it used to and you have fluid backing up into your lungs, which is causing you to feel short of breath" be more appropriate? Remember that people tend to only remember about 10% of what their providers tell them. Make it as easy as possible for them to do that. Draw pictures if you need to.

Listen to what patients and families have to say. They usually have unique insight into what is going on with the patient. Do not discount their input.

See your patients with your preceptors, even if you saw them on your own already. Watching your preceptor interact with patients and their families is invaluable. You can learn new ways to interview, see demonstrations of physical exam techniques and findings and observe how your preceptor puts a scared kid at ease, talks down an irate family member or treats the hungry homeless guy who really just wants to get out of the cold for a couple of hours with kindness and respect.

You will encounter patients and families of patients who frustrate you or who make decisions that you disagree with. Be mindful of your body language, tone and facial expressions and remember that this is not about you. We all have different values, perspectives, and cultural beliefs. Our jobs as providers is to present all of the possible options and best recommendations in an objective manner to help patients and families make informed decisions that align with their belief systems. Keep your personal opinions to yourself, keep your cool and do not get involved in any drama. Excuse yourself and step out, if necessary.

Helpful hint: If your patient has alarming symptoms or appears to be decompensating, go get your preceptor right away.

Invest In Your Experience

Be an active participant in your learning and be eager to learn whatever your preceptor is willing to teach you. Let your preceptor know if there is something in particular that you want to learn or try. If appropriate, he or she will more than likely try to arrange it for you.

Be the kind of student who is just as excited to suture her 100th laceration as she was her first. Be the kind of student who recognizes that there is something to learn from each and every patient interaction. Even if you've done 500 well baby exams (I exaggerate), know that there is something to learn from number 501.

 Scrub in for your 10th lap choley of the day? You bet!

Stay late for that family meeting? Of course.

Replace the NG tube that you just placed and the patient just pulled? On it!

Spend the day in pre-op putting in IV's? Yes, please!

Want to come down to the lab with me to look at this smear? Absolutely!

Stay well past the end of your shift to help manage your unstable patient? No place else I'd rather be.

Never, ever be the kind of student who says, "I don't need to learn that" or "I already know how to do that". And don't be the student who hides away in the corner, eyes glued to her phone, head stuck in a book or who disappears when there is work to be done.

Surgical Rotations

Surgery is a different breed than medicine. There are some extra things you should know about your surgical rotation.

Before the OR

Earlier, we touched on scrubbing into the OR. Practice this before your rotation starts. Know how to scrub and know how to gown. The scrub nurse will not let you in her OR if she thinks that you will compromise sterility.

Know your glove size and practice, practice, practice putting them on. Struggling to get your gloves on is embarrassing. Trust me, I know.

Know how to properly de-gown and de-glove so that you don't get anything on you that you really don't want to get on you. Make sure that you throw away your own trash. Do not leave your garbage on the floor.

Get familiar with common surgical instruments. Know the difference between a Kelly clamp and forceps and practice handling them, just in case you get to use them.

Know how to suture and know how to tie a suture. My first rotation was OB/GYN. I foolishly did not practice suture tying before that rotation and it came back to bite me. The attending physician allowed me to deliver a baby on my own, which was an amazing, incredible, wonderful experience. The patient had a tear, however, that needed suturing and I did not know how to hand tie. I simply did not practice it and could not remember how to do it. I cannot tell you how bad it felt to see the look of disappointment on the attending's face when I told him that I wasn't sure what to do. I got pushed aside and got knocked down a peg. Don't put yourself in that position. Put the time in and get to practicing. Make sure that you know how to both instrument tie and hand tie. Know when is best to use each type of stitch and know when to use which type of suture material. You will learn about all of this in your didactic surgery unit. If it's not covered, be sure to ask about it.

Surgeons love to pimp, meaning that they love to quiz your knowledge, especially your knowledge of anatomy and pathophysiology, as well as indications for surgeries and complications for certain surgical procedures. Don't let this make you nervous. Just anticipate it and prepare for it. Will you know every answer? Of course not. But, showing effort goes a long way. And you already know what to do if you don't know the answer, right?

Try to figure out what cases you will be in and prep for them. Review the anatomy, including blood supply to the area that is being operated on and familiarize yourself with the procedure itself. Many students love the book <u>Surgical Recall</u>.

Wear comfortable shoes. You might be on your feet for hours on end in the OR or you may be scurrying around trying to keep up with the team during rounds. Heels are not your friend here.

Trim your nails and take off your nail polish. At our program, we make everyone remove their acrylics and gels. Some OR's won't let you in if your nails are not short and natural.

Remove your jewelry, especially rings and bracelets. Some people put their rings on a necklace, but I just left mine at home. I got engaged just before PA school started, so I loved wearing my engagement ring, but I was too scared that I would lose it if I wore it around my neck. Do what you feel most comfortable doing.

In the OR

Sterility is the name of the game in the OR.

Tuck away your lanyard or name badge before scrubbing. Loose items easily contaminate your hands while bending over to scrub.

Always put on your booties, cap, and mask before entering the OR. You need these in place before you gown and glove because they are dirty.

Once gowned and gloved, be mindful of where your hands are. Keep your hands above your waist. Anything below the waist is not sterile. Don't touch your head, neck, or face. They are not sterile. Don't put your hands on your hips. Your back and sides are not sterile. If something falls, let it fall because, you guessed it, it is no longer sterile. Basically, stand there with your hands clasped in front of your chest, waiting for instruction. Sometimes you will just observe, other times you will hold the retractor and, if you are lucky, you'll get to do some other stuff, too.

Never touch anything you do not have expressed permission to touch. Ever. More than likely, you will find yourself positioned next to the scrub tech and his or her tray. Do not touch that tray. Do not take instruments off of the tray and do not pass instruments from the scrub tech to the surgeon unless you are asked to do so. Mishandling of instruments can result in injury. You don't want to be the one who accidentally stabbed the surgeon with the scalpel, do you? If you do have permission to receive and pass instruments, do so politely.

Watch where you are walking. There are plenty of wires, tubes, pedals, and whatnot to trip over. If you trip, you can fall into the sterile field. Try not to do that.

The circulator nurse will be watching you like a hawk. She will notice if you break sterility and she will call you out on it. Loudly, probably, and most likely in an annoyed tone. Thank her for letting you know and then go change your gloves or whatever else needs changing so that you can get back in there.

If you happen to break sterility by even just barely grazing an unsterile surface with your gloved hand and no one notices but you, make sure that you call yourself out. Tell the circulator that you broke sterility and need to gown and glove again. Is it embarrassing? Yup, it sure is. But guess what? Everyone has done it at one point or another, probably multiple times. It happens. Honestly, you will gain the respect of the OR staff if you admit that you made a mistake because doing so shows that you value the safety of the patient and that you respect the OR and its team.

Speaking of safety ... if you start to feel woozy, tell someone that you are feeling unwell and step away from the sterile field. To avoid passing out in the OR, make sure that you are well hydrated and have a little something in your belly before you walk through the doors. I almost passed out once, but as soon as I felt that feeling coming on, I expressed it out loud and stepped away from the table. The nurse escorted me out of the OR, helped me get out of my gown, had me sit down and gave me some apple juice. I felt better after a couple of minutes and I asked for permission to get back in there. I was a little embarrassed, but that little bit of embarrassment is so much better than how I would have felt if I had passed out into the sterile field.

Be safe

Personal Safety

There are instances when patients and families get violent. Situations in which this is more likely to occur include when someone is intoxicated or high, when there is mental instability, when emotions or tensions are high, when you are denying someone something that they want or when you are delivering bad news. Sometimes the threat is obvious like when, for example, the guy is wheeled in kicking and screaming, "I am going to kill you all!". But, other times the signs can be more subtle. We had a resident who was punched in the face by a family member after she told her that her husband had passed away. Believe me, she was not expecting that reaction. Watch for signs of escalation such as increased agitation, raising of the voice, pacing, quick, short words, etc. Make sure that you maintain your personal space and trust your instincts. Always make sure that you have a clear path to the door, even in low-risk situations. Maneuver around people if that's what it takes to keep that path clear. If it is the patient who is the potential threat, make sure that you can move away quickly, if necessary. Be mindful of where the patient's hands are in relation to you, even if they are restrained, and keep your hands and face away from their mouth. Don't be afraid to call for help or to ask the nurse to be there with you.

I always tell patients what I am about to do or ask permission to do it so that they are not surprised by my movement or touch. "Mr. Jones, I am going to listen to your heart now. Is that ok?". This is especially important with potentially violent patients and unstable psychiatric patients. If you feel uncomfortable going in alone to see a patient, don't. Trust your gut. We subconsciously pick up on stuff well before we consciously process it. Ask your preceptor to see the patient with you. If you feel weird about this, phrase your request in such a way that it sounds like you are interested in learning how to best deal with the situation. Not only will doing that make you feel safer, but it gives you the opportunity to see how a more seasoned provider handles it. Be proactive about your safety. There are no do-overs.

If you are on rotation at a hospital and are leaving late at night, ask security to give you a ride to your car. That is part of their job, it is what they are there for and they are more than happy to do it.

If you ever feel threatened or harassed while on rotation by your preceptor, staff members, students, or anyone else, tell your clinical director right away. Programs should not tolerate that kind of behavior.

Other Safety Considerations

Sharps – make sure that you are handling sharps properly. Do not recap needles. Do not shove your hand into a sharps container. Always be mindful of where your sharps are when you are doing a procedure and be careful of your sharps when you are cleaning up from a procedure. Discard of them first. If you get stuck, tell your preceptor right away, let your clinical director know and follow the protocols at the site and those set forth by your program.

Isolation precautions – always wear the proper PPE (personal protective equipment). Make sure you check to see if someone is on precautions and what PPE is necessary before you go into a patient room. Always wash your hands or use hand sanitizer before and after patient encounters. FYI: hand washing, rather than hand sanitizing, is required for patients with c. diff.

Radiology suite – use proper shielding, step as far away from the source as possible and listen to the radiology staff. Be extra cautious if you are pregnant. Never enter an MRI room unless you have express permission to do so. Follow the instructions given to you at that time. Those magnets are super powerful. People have died.

Helpful hint: although this isn't a safety issue per say, make sure that you eat and stay well hydrated. Keep a protein bar in your pocket and tuck a water bottle into the break room. If you are on an inpatient rotation, go to lunch rounds. You will learn something interesting and they will feed you, too!

Hipaa (Health Insurance Portability And Accountability Act Of 1996) Compliance

Remember how I mentioned earlier that we enter a contract of trust with our patients when we take care of them? Being compliant with HIPAA is one of the parameters of that trust. HIPAA is a federal law that was created to ensure that patients' personal information is protected. This means that we cannot disclosed that information without the consent or knowledge of the patient. That means that we are not allowed to discuss any part of the patient's care with anyone without the patient saying that it is ok to do so. Patients fill out paperwork that lets their healthcare providers know what information may be disclosed and to whom it may be disclosed. A caveat to this pertains to medical staff. You do not need to ask the patient if it is ok for you to review their chart if they come to see you. It is understood that you will review their medical records in order to take care of them. It is also understood that you will discuss details of the patient's case with other healthcare workers, such as nurses, CNA's, consultants, and your preceptor. But, be careful of what you say and where you say it. It is inappropriate to discuss patients in the elevator, in line at the cafeteria, while standing around in crowed or busy hallways or in any other space where what you are saying can be overheard by someone not involved in the case. You should only review the charts of patients for whom you are directly caring or patients being cared for by your team in the hospital setting, for example.

Let's go through a couple of scenarios:

Your friend's dad has been admitted to the hospital. You are not at all involved in his care. Can you review his chart and let your friend know what is going on? No. Only open charts in which you or you care team are directly involved.

Can you snoop through the chart of the celebrity who is in the emergency department? You swear you won't tell anyone anything that you found. No, doing so is a HIPAA violation.

Can you look through your own records? No, most institutions do now allow you to look up your own information.

A family member calls asking for an update about your patient, but his name is not on the list of contacts. The patient is intubated and sedated and cannot speak for herself. Can you provide an update? No, you may not provide any details of the patient's care to that caller because his name is not on the contact list. Always make sure that you know the name of the person you are talking to and check to see if that name is on the approved contact list. If so, fill them in. If not, politely tell them that you are not allowed to provide any information, as they are not on the list.

What if the family member insists that he should be on the list? Politely advise the family member to get in touch with the designated healthcare representative (should be listed in the computer as the primary contact person) who can then call the hospital and update the list with his name.

What if family is at bedside and is requesting an update for an unresponsive or confused patient? Again, know your audience. Politely introduce yourself and ask with whom you are speaking. If the healthcare representative is among the group, provide the update. If no one in the room is on the contact list, provide very general information and advise them to get in touch with the healthcare representative if they want more detailed answers. This differs from a telephone update in that the people requesting the update are in the room, so they clearly know something about the patient's care.

What if family is at bedside and the patient is awake and interactive? Directly ask the patient if it is ok to provide an update. If so, go for it. If not, politely let the family members know that you must respect your patient's wishes.

What if my patient, who has HIV tells you not to disclose her HIV status to her husband with whom she is actively sexually active. Can I tell her husband? What if I feel like he has the right to know? It is a HIPAA violation to disclose any information that the patient does not want you to disclose, no matter how unfair that may seem.

A father of an 18-year-old patient called to ask if that patient had an abortion at our clinic. She is covered under his insurance. What do I tell him? As she is 18 years old, she is an adult and so her information is protected under HIPAA. Unless she gave permission to disclose that information to her father, doing so would be a HIPAA violation.

What if, in that same scenario, the patient was 16 years old? It depends upon the situation. You would need to gather more information to make your decision.

If you encounter any situations such as these or if you are ever unsure of what the right thing to do is, put the caller on hold or excuse yourself from the room and ask your preceptor for guidance.

Helpful hint: Don't post details on social media about your clinical experiences. Even if you don't use names or mention the site, sometimes a description of what happened, especially if it is an unusual or unique circumstance, can be a HIPPA violation. Don't talk trash about your preceptor, staff, the site, or patients. Not only can it hurt you in the here and now, but derogatory posts can also hurt your future employment prospects.

Documentation

If you don't document it, it never happened.

Patients have access to their medical records, often in real time. Be careful with your wording and the tone of your note.

Studying During Clinicals

When your shift is over, go home and read, read, read. This will take some discipline on your part because you have a lot more freedom in clinical year. Once you walk off the site, what you do with your time is entirely up to you. Remember that you are still in school, though, and that you still have to pass an end-of-rotation exam. In terms of study techniques, you should have a pretty good idea of what works for you by this time. Some students like to Rosh Review, Smarty PANCE or other exam review materials. However you choose to study, do it consistently.

Call Back

At the end of each clinical rotation, you will head back to campus for your end-of-rotation exams (EOR's). This could include a multiple choice exam, an OSCE, demonstration of an associated clinical procedure or any combination of the above. Your program will let you know what is expected of you for the EOR's. You should, of course, be prepared for your exam. But beyond that, have fun. Catch up with your classmates, swap stories, share what you've learned and enjoy being together again. Most programs require that you participate in grand rounds, which is an opportunity for you to formally present an interesting patient case and explain a clinical concept in the context of that case. Grand rounds is usually scheduled during call back after exams. Your clinical director will let you know in advance when you are scheduled to present. If it is your turn, take pride in being the expert in the room for your particular topic and if you are in the audience, ask great questions and draw connections to your own experiences. I loved attending my students' grand rounds. I learned a lot of interesting stuff and I felt like a proud Mama sitting there watching my students grow and flourish right before my eyes.

EARNING YOUR MASTER'S

As of this writing, the master's degree is the terminal degree for physician assistants.

So how do you earn your master's degree? Some programs require that you write a thesis, others a capstone project and yet others will require you to pass comprehensive written, practical, and oral examinations. Take this into consideration when choosing a program.

Capstone

The Capstone project is a year-long research project that usually begins in the second year of school. Basically, you start by asking questions about a topic of interest to you. Some programs require you to tie your question to a clinical case you saw on rotation, while some do not. Once you have what you think is a good question, you present it to your advisor who will either accept it, reject it, or ask you to refine it. Then, you get to researching. Most programs require that a certain percentage of your research material is from academic journal articles that were written within a certain time period. Typically, you will have deadlines along the way and will receive feedback for what you are submitting. Most programs require the creation of a summary poster and some require a formal oral presentation. Your program will provide you with instructions and guidance.

Thesis

The thesis is similar to the Capstone project in that you answer a clinical question by performing extensive research. Again, you will work closely with your advisor and you will be required to present your thesis to a committee for scoring.

The goal of both the Capstone project and the thesis is to get you comfortable with researching, reading, and interpreting clinical literature. Publication is a possible outcome.

I'VE GRADUATED. NOW WHAT?

Now that you have graduated, you can join the National Commission on Certification of Physician Assistants (NCCPA), which is the national credentialing board for physician assistants and then to take the PANCE. The PANCE is a 300-question test that is administered in five 60-minute blocks, each of which consists of 60 questions. Most students have already joined the NCCPA and scheduled their testing session prior to graduation. Some students already have their CV already to go and some students have already interviewed and accepted jobs. Wherever you are in this process is just fine. You will all eventually get to the same place: employment as a PA-C.

Studying for the pance

Most students study for the PANCE by doing review questions over and over and over again. Rosh Review, Smarty PANCE and PANCE Pre Pearls are popular choices. Make sure that you check out the NCCPA website, as it has a lot of good information about the PANCE. The blueprint provides an excellent overview of what is covered on the exam.

Credentialing

Once you pass your PANCE and are designated Physician Assistant – Certified (woo-hoo!!!), you can apply for state licensure. Additionally, you will need to obtain your Drug Enforcement

Agency (DEA) certificate to prescribe medications and your state certificate for controlled substances, if required. Check with the guidelines for the state where you will be working for specifics. If you work in multiple states, you will need to obtain licensure in each state and if you work in multiple hospitals, you will need to undergo the credentialing process for each hospital.

Ongoing requirements

In order to remain in good standing with the NCCPA, you will need to complete 100 hours of Continuing Medical Education (CME) hours within a two-year period. Physician assistants are required to recertify by taking the Physician Assistant National Recertifying Exam (PANRE) every 10 years. Please see the NCCPA website at www.NCCPA.net for further details about CME requirements and recertification.

Finding a job

More often than not, what you thought you wanted to do when you got into PA school is different than what you decide you want to do upon graduation. I, for example, thought I wanted to work in emergency medicine. I liked the idea of the patient acuity, of working in a buzzing, bustling emergency department, saving lives and all that good stuff. But, my ED rotation was my least favorite. I did like the acuity and I did like the variety, but the pace and the fleetingness of patient interactions didn't appeal to me. When I did my internal medicine rotation, however, it was like the heavens opened up and the angels sang. I knew I was home. I loved the detail-oriented nature of internal medicine. I loved crossing all the T's and dotting all of the I's. I loved talking with the patients and their families, eliciting all of their medical history, social history, work history. But what I liked the most was the day-to-day care of the patient. I liked getting to know the patients and their families.

I really enjoyed seeing how each day unfolded and what we could do to make it better. I liked the critical thinking and the prolonged patient interaction.

Maybe your rotations will confirm your initial ideas, maybe you will have an epiphany moment like I did, or maybe you will graduate PA school with no idea what you want to do. What if, in the end, you were no more certain of what you wanted to do than when you started PA school? That's ok. Not knowing exactly what you want to do is actually quite common. If that is the case, then perhaps working in a generalized discipline like internal med, primary care or general surgery would be helpful so that you can figure out what it is that you really love.

Go back to when you decided that you wanted to be a PA. What did you envision? How did you feel? Did you want to save lives by revascularizing coronary arteries in the cath lab or did you see yourself making sure that you improved the quality of your patient's lives by being a mental health provider? Go back to the beginning and re-identify with what made you want to be a PA the first place. And then take some time to think about which rotations you really liked, which ones were just kind of meh and which, if any, you did not particularly enjoy. Figure out what it was about each that you liked or disliked, compile a list of "what I want" for a job and go figure out which discipline best fits that list. Take scheduling into consideration, as well. If you do not want to work nights, weekends, and holidays, then a job in the hospital is not a good fit. If you want to work three twelve hour shifts instead of five eight-hour shifts, then primary care is not a good fit.

Next, do a self-inventory. What were you good at on your rotations? What were you not good at? Were you a superstar at suturing or did your sewing look like Dr Frankenstein did it? Were your oral presentations eloquent and seamless? Were you a diagnostic whiz? Figure out what you were good at and where you could best use your attributes.

As I mentioned, I loved my internal medicine rotation, so internal medicine was a natural choice for me. And I loved it. They were my people. As I gained more and more experience, I was able to further identify and delineate just what I did and did not like. For example, I found little satisfaction in admitting the 98-year-old ladies with the "dwindles" who took 45 medications and had a past medical history the length of my arm. Mind you, I still took excellent care of these patients, appreciated the privilege of taking care of them and went over their charts and histories with a fine-tooth comb, but they were not my favorite patient population. What I did love, however, were the critically ill patients who we admitted to the ICU. I loved how complicated they were, how much they made me think. I loved that multiple organ systems were involve with their illnesses and I loved trying to figure out how it all went together. I loved solving the puzzle, or at least trying to solve it. So, after many years as a hospitalist, I took the leap and transitioned to critical care. That's one of the great things about being a PA. When and if you are ready to switch disciplines, you can.

Pay off my loans?

PA school is expensive, no doubt. But, we get paid pretty well. So, if you are able to live at home for a bit or continue to share an apartment with roommates, you can use the majority of your extra income to pay down your student loan debt. If that isn't your thing, there are programs out there that will pay off your student loans if you commit to working with them for a certain number of years. These programs typically focus on serving underprivileged communities – practical and noble. Otherwise, make your monthly payments and throw an extra couple of bucks at them every now and then.

Resources

National Commission on Certification of Physician Assistants (NCCPA)

(this is where you sign up for the PANCE and PANRE and also

where you log all of your CME)

American Association of Physician Assistants (AAPA)
(this is the professional society for physician assistants)

Physician Assistant Education Association (PAEA)
(this organization represents PA education programs)

Supplemental materials for studying

Here is a list of some of the most frequently recommended online and paperback sources for supplemental study:

American Academy of Family Physicians (AAFP) website – this website has a lot of nice charts and tables and explains complex medical issues very well. I actually used this site a lot as a reference when preparing lectures.

Epocrates – provides medication information

ExamMaster – exam prep and practice

HippoEd – exam prep and practice, explainer videos

OnlineMedEd – explainer videos

Osmosis Med – exam prep and explainer videos

MedCram – explainer videos

NCCPA blueprint – overview of what is on the PANCE

PAEA blueprint and topic list – overview of what is on the PANCE

PANCE Pre Pearls – exam prep and review

Rosh Review – exam prep and review

Smarty PANCE and Rotation Exam Review – exam prep and review

Step Up to Medicine – medicine review

Quizlet – virtual flash cards

Up-To-Date – online reference resource

CONCLUSION

You are joining one of the best professions out there. It is a rewarding, challenging, fulfilling and meaningful career. I wish you all the best and hope to see you out there in the clinical world!! Thank you for allowing me to share a little bit of what I know with you!!

Made in United States
Troutdale, OR
09/18/2023